Venepuncture and
Cannulation

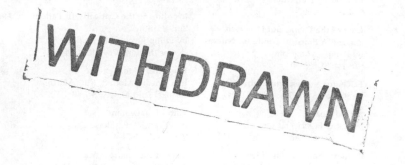

Essential Clinical Skills for Nurses

The *Essential Clinical Skills for Nurses* series focuses on key clinical skills for nurses and other health professionals. These concise, accessible books assume no prior knowledge and focus on core clinical skills, clearly presenting common clinical procedures and their rationale, together with the essential background theory. Their user-friendly format makes them an indispensable guide to clinical practice for all nurses, especially to student nurses and newly qualified staff.

Other titles in the *Essential Clinical Skills for Nurses* series:

Venepuncture and Cannulation

Edited by

Sarah Phillips
Education and Organisation Consultant,
Vein Train Ltd

Mary Collins
Clinical Practice Educator, Imperial College
Healthcare NHS Trust

Lisa Dougherty, OBE
Nurse Consultant Intravenous Therapy, The Royal
Marsden Hospital NHS Foundation Trust

WILEY-BLACKWELL

A John Wiley & Sons, Ltd., Publication

This edition first published 2011. © 2011 by Blackwell Publishing Ltd

Blackwell Publishing was acquired by John Wiley & Sons in February 2007. Blackwell's publishing program has been merged with Wiley's global Scientific, Technical and Medical business to form Wiley-Blackwell.

Registered office: John Wiley & Sons Ltd, The Atrium, Southern Gate, Chichester, West Sussex, PO19 8SQ, UK

Editorial offices: 9600 Garsington Road, Oxford, OX4 2DQ, UK
2121 State Avenue, Ames, Iowa 50014-8300, USA

For details of our global editorial offices, for customer services and for information about how to apply for permission to reuse the copyright material in this book please see our website at www.wiley.com/wiley-blackwell.

The right of the author to be identified as the author of this work has been asserted in accordance with the UK Copyright, Designs and Patents Act 1988.

Library of Congress Cataloging-in-Publication Data

Venepuncture and cannulation / edited by Sarah Phillips, Mary Collins, Lisa Dougherty.
    p. ; cm. – (Essential clinical skills for nurses)
  Includes bibliographical references and index.
  ISBN 978-1-4051-4860-3 (pbk. : alk. paper)
1. Veins–Puncture. 2. Catheterization. 3. Nursing. I. Phillips, Sarah, 1972- II. Collins, Mary, 1971- III. Dougherty, Lisa. IV. Series: Essential clinical skills for nurses.
  [DNLM: 1. Phlebotomy–nursing. 2. Catheterization–nursing. WY 100.1] RM182.V46 2011
  615'.39–dc22

                              2010041325

A catalogue record for this book is available from the British Library.

This book is published in the following electronic formats: ePDF 9781444393217; Wiley Online Library 9781444393231; ePub 9781444393224

Set in 9/11 pt Palatino by Toppan Best-set Premedia Limited
Printed and bound in Malaysia by Vivar Printing Sdn Bhd

1 2011

Contents

Foreword

Venepuncture and cannulation are two commonly practiced invasive procedures in the hospital and community setting that have remained unchanged despite technological developments of the past decades. These are not complex procedures, however there are a number of factors that contribute to correctly performing them, presented by the authors in this book.

The wide variety of clinicians offering these skills to their patients is welcome and makes the most of the talent in the NHS, while offering patients choice and an efficient service. However, such diversity risks different types of practices evolving. It is therefore essential that a clear, concise yet informative text is available for clinicians to lead forward best practice in the most appropriate and informative way.

The book provides a comprehensive yet concise overview of relevant information and assumes no specialist knowledge. The text is augmented by useful tables and diagrams and is logically presented for reading and reference purposes. Competent practice and patient experience are integrated throughout with additional designated chapters from both the patient perspective and the educational experience. This demonstrates the editors' commitment to providing a text with a strong emphasis on high quality patient care, and the importance of training and education in order to achieve that aim. All relevant aspects are covered, beginning with professionals, and their duty of care and legal responsibilities. The book is completed by a review of the patient experience, specifically what we know about their experience and how this can shape our practice.

I welcome this book as the first publication on venepuncture and cannulation in the United Kingdom. It is further example of how the NHS in particular, remains at the forefront of pioneering clinical practice development in healthcare worldwide.

Expertise, patient experience and evidence based practice are shared by texts like this to ensure practising clinicians may take available knowledge and skill forward and continue to offer a first class service for our patients.

Venepuncture and Cannulation – Essential Clinical Skills for Nurses, provides a core text for anyone practicing these skills, not just nurses. The extensive referencing and content from authors, with both expertise and knowledge in this field, make this book both an excellent starting and reference point. It will become a pivotal reference for the clinician who strives to master, rather than simply acquire these skills.

Professor Lord Darzi PC, KBE, FMedSci, HonFREng

Professor Darzi holds the Paul Hamlyn Chair of Surgery at Imperial College London where he is Head of Division of Surgery. He is internationally respected for his innovative work in the advancement of minimal invasive surgery and the development and use of allied technologies. Research led by Professor Darzi is directed towards achieving best surgical practice through both innovation in surgery and enhancing the safety and quality of healthcare.

Contributors

Andrea Blay Consultant Nurse Critical Care, Chelsea and Westminster Hospital NHS Foundation Trust

Mary Collins Clinical Practice Educator, Imperial College Healthcare NHS Trust

Annie de Verteuil Senior Clinical Skills Trainer, Royal Berkshire NHS Foundation Trust

Mirjana Dojcinovska ST2 Respiratory Medicine, Papworth Hospital NHS Foundation Trust

Lisa Dougherty OBE Nurse Consultant Intravenous Therapy, The Royal Marsden NHS Foundation Trust

Sarah Hart Formerly Clinical Nurse Specialist Infection Control, The Royal Marsden Hospital NHS Foundation Trust

Lorraine Hyde Matron Day Services, The Royal Marsden Hospital NHS Foundation Trust

Wendy Morris Infection Prevention and Control Nurse, Royal Berkshire NHS Foundation Trust

Sarah Phillips Education and Organisation Consultant, Vein Train Ltd

Barbara Witt Nurse Phlebotomist, The Royal Marsden Hospital NHS Foundation Trust

Introduction

Sarah Phillips and Mary Collins

This book aims to equip healthcare practitioners with underlying theory prior to gaining competence in the hospital and community settings for the practical skills of venepuncture and cannulation. It is predicted that users of this book are the practitioner who is updating their knowledge about these skills or the novice who is learning the skill of venepuncture or cannulation for the first time before undertaking supervised practice in the clinical environment.

Intravenous access is a skill that is growing amongst all healthcare practitioners and there are a number of reasons why it is required:

1. Administration of 'short-term low-risk intravenous therapy e.g. administration of blood and blood produces, isotonic fluids and drugs whose pH and osmolarity are similar to that of blood' (Scales 2005, p. 48).
2. New roles and autonomy for community nurses (Maben & Griffiths 2008, p. 13).
3. Nurses responsible for the management of whole episodes of care for patients (Maben & Griffiths 2008, p. 13).
4. Provision of 'safe, effective and prompt nursing interventions' a core element of good quality nursing care (Maben & Griffiths 2008).
5. The Hospital at Night (HaN) concept is one such example to achieve seamless clinical care with one or more multiprofessional teams who between them have the full range of skills and competencies to meet patients' immediate needs.

Venepuncture and Cannulation, first edition. Edited by Sarah Phillips,
Mary Collins and Lisa Dougherty. Published 2011 by Blackwell Publishing Ltd.
© 2011 Blackwell Publishing Ltd.

The chapters individually highlight good practice, and therefore quality care, in the stages that collectively ensure the patient's safety throughout the procedure of venepuncture and cannulation. This is pertinent in light of the current agenda that focuses on quality outlined in the Darzi report *High Quality Care for All* (2008a). This report places emphasis on achieving effective and high quality healthcare services by enabling practitioners to utilise their skills, knowledge and expertise appropriately and effectively. 'NHS staff make the difference where it matters most and we have an obligation to patients and the public to enable them to make best use of their talents' (Darzi 2008a, p. 10).

The authors of this book consider education and training to be pivotal in providing best practice for patients in these skills. It is equally recognised that achieving this basic requirement is challenging for practitioners and managers in today's fast moving healthcare. The following recommendations offer a realistic way forward in modern healthcare and are echoed throughout this book:

- Flexible – provision of education and training must be sufficiently flexible to give professionals both the breadth and depth of expertise that they need to deliver the high quality care to which they aspire
- Focused on quality – high quality care requires the provision of high quality education and training
- Promoting life-long learning: Staff in all roles and settings need opportunities to continuously update the skills and techniques that are relevant to delivering high quality care through, for example, work-based learning. ...

Darzi (2008b, p. 12)

For the purpose of the book the practitioner refers to anyone who is undertaking the skills of venepuncture and cannulation. This can be a healthcare assistant, phlebotomist, physician's assistant, medical student, registered nurse, midwife, qualified doctor or radiographer. References are made to paediatrics; however, this book is focused on cannulation and venepuncture for the adult or adolescent.

Chapter 1 considers *the legal and professional aspects* which the practitioner must familiarise themselves with prior to undertaking *the learning experience*, which is the focus of Chapter 2. Preparing for these procedures requires some specific knowledge and understanding, therefore *anatomy and physiology* is covered in Chapter 3 and *selecting the correct equipment*, for example blood bottles, cannulae, for the procedure in Chapter 4. A particularly important consideration for the success of these procedures is to ensure that the patient has the best experience possible. This means *selecting the correct vein* is crucial and Chapter 5 looks at assessing the patient, inspection and palpation of the vein, and considers some challenges that the practitioner may encounter. In view of the increasing numbers of intravascular catheter-related bloodstream infections, Chapter 6 addresses *infection control and risk management*. Preparation of both the patient and the practitioner increases the success of these procedures and these are considered in Chapter 7 in *procedures for venepuncture and cannulation*. Complications are a reality and Chapter 8 helps the practitioner to identify when they occur and problem-solve to minimise injury for the patient. Chapter 9 covers *different types of blood tests* and factors that must be considered when taking blood. Finally, central to the success of these procedures is the patient and their perspectives are addressed in Chapter 10.

SOME DEFINITIONS OF COMMON TERMS USED IN THIS BOOK

Cannulation: The 'insertion of a tube into a body duct or cavity, is performed to provide access to the circulation for the administration of short-term, low-risk intravenous therapy' (Scales 2005, p. 48).

Venepuncture: The term used to describe the procedure of 'Entering a vein with a needle' (Dougherty & Lister 2011, p. 920).

REFERENCES
Darzi, A.W. (2008a) *High Quality Care For All: NHS Next Stage Review Final Report*. DH, London.
Darzi, A.W. (2008b) *A High Quality Workforce. NHS Next Stage Review*. DH, London.

Dougherty, L. & Lister, S. (2011) *The Royal Marsden Hospital Manual of Clinical Nursing Procedures*, 8th edn. Wiley Blackwell, Oxford.

Maben, J. & Griffiths, P. (2008) *Nurses in Society: Starting the Debate*. National Nursing Research Unit King's College London, London.

Scales, K. (2005) Vascular access: a guide to peripheral venous cannulation. *Nursing Standard*, **19**(49), 48–52.

Legal and Professional Issues

1

Lorraine Hyde

LEARNING OUTCOMES

The practitioner will be able to:

- ❏ Understand key aspects of the legal framework that are relevant to these skills.
- ❏ Understand how healthcare organisations operate within this framework, in relation to these skills.
- ❏ Consider the professional aspects for these skills.
- ❏ Understand the importance of evidence-based practice.

INTRODUCTION

Venepuncture and cannulation are the most commonly performed invasive procedures in the NHS. To perform these procedures well, and to ensure a satisfactory outcome for the patient, requires the practitioner to have relevant and up-to-date knowledge and skill (Dougherty 2008). This chapter focuses on the legal and professional implications for nurses who perform these procedures within their practice setting.

THE LEGAL ASPECT

The nursing profession seeks to deliver high quality care at all times and the role of the nurse has expanded significantly over the past decade. The evolving range of responsibilities can be

---

Venepuncture and Cannulation, first edition. Edited by Sarah Phillips,
Mary Collins and Lisa Dougherty. Published 2011 by Blackwell Publishing Ltd.
© 2011 Blackwell Publishing Ltd.

complex in nature and are related to the technological and medical advances within the healthcare setting. The nurse's role, whilst offering intellectual stimulation and professional satisfaction, brings with it the potential for increased legal risks (Hyde 2008). Nurses must have a working knowledge of the law and how it applies to their practice in order to be safe and competent practitioners.

Sources of law

The law derives from two main sources. The first is Acts of Parliament and Statutory Instruments (also known as statute law) which are enabled by the powers given to Parliament (Hyde 2008). These statutes, which take precedence over all other laws, include the legislation of the European Community. Laws of the European Community automatically become part of the law in the United Kingdom (Dimond 2005). There are many statutes that apply to nursing, such as the Nurses Midwives and Health Visitors Act 1997, the National Health Service Act 1977 and the Health Act 1999.

The common law (also known as case law) is the second source, which is derived from decisions made by judges in individual cases. Thus, common law operates through a system of precedent. The judge, when considering the facts before him and deciding upon a case, is bound by the decision in law made by judges at an earlier case if it is relevant to the facts before him and if that decision was made by a higher court to that in which he is sitting (Dimond 2005). The established order of precedence means that decisions made in the United Kingdom Supreme Court, the highest court of the land, are binding over all lower courts except itself, but would be subject to relevant precedents established in the European Court of Justice (Dimond 2005).

The legal system is divided into two main branches, criminal and civil law. Criminal law relates to crime and breaches can lead to prosecution, whilst civil law deals with all other cases (Hodgson 2002). Civil law is the branch of law whereby a civil action for negligence in relation to the liability of the nurse would be heard. A patient who has suffered harm as a consequence of inadequate care whilst being treated by the nurse can claim compensation for a breach of duty of care. It is therefore important that the nurse has an understanding of liability in relation to civil action.

THE PROFESSIONAL ASPECT

Statutory regulation of nurses is the function of the Nursing and Midwifery Council (NMC). The professional register is a means of declaring that a reasonable standard of competence and conduct is expected from those named in it. It is also stating that these are the people to whom the NMC has declared its expectations, given its advice and presented its standards, and to whom it can call to account. The Nursing Midwifery Order 2001 requires the NMC to have specific statutory committees, these are the:

- Screeners and Practice Committees – who consider allegation and establish if the complaint is well founded but who may refer the matter to the other committee for consideration
- Investigating Committee (IC)
- Conduct and Competence Committee (CCC)
- Health Committee (HC).

Integral to the NMC function is to protect the public from persons whose fitness to practise is impaired. Fitness to practise implies the registrant's suitability to be on the register without restrictions. Some of the ways in which fitness to practise may be impaired are by misconduct, lack of competence, physical or mental ill-health or a criminal conviction. The CCC holds hearings in public to encourage transparency and to reflect the NMC's public accountability. The sanctions that are available to the committees include issuing a caution, suspension from the register or removal from the register. As a way of ensuring that practitioners are fit to practise and are able to provide relevant and evidence-based nursing intervention, the NMC provides guidance through its Code, which was updated in April 2008. It states: 'The people in your care must be able to trust you with their health and wellbeing', and it requires the nurse or midwife to:

 – make the care of people your first concern, treating them as individuals and respecting their dignity

- work with others to protect and promote the health and well-being of those in your care, their families and carers, and the wider community
- provide a high standard of practice and care at all times
- be open and honest, act with integrity and uphold the reputation of your profession.

NMC (2008) p. 1

ACCOUNTABILITY

The concept of accountability is influenced by issues such as authority and autonomy and is related to the concept of professionalism. Watson (2004) states that 'accountability is the hallmark of a profession' in that training and professional registration is required in order to practise. The nurse has both professional and legal accountability for her practice. Nurses are accountable to:

- the NMC in terms of the code of conduct, and the sanction could be removal from the register
- the patient through civil law, and the sanction could be to be sued by the patient
- the employer through contract of employment/employment tribunal, and sanction could be loss of job
- the public through criminal law/courts, and the sanction could be criminal prosecution (Hyde 2008).

There can be overlap within these areas of accountability. For example, if a nurse witnesses a car accident, legally she is not obliged to stop at the scene and offer assistance; however, professionally she would be expected to. The NMC states that the nurse is 'accountable for the care she delivers in emergency situations'.

Accountability is implicit within any area of practice where the practitioner is delivering care. The NMC defines accountability as 'responsible for something or someone', and to be responsible requires knowledge. Clark (2000) describes accountability as meaning 'the professional takes a decision or action not because someone has told him or her to do so, but because, having weighed up the alternatives and consequences in the light of the best available knowledge, he or she believes it is the right decision or action to take'. The NMC states that in exercising their professional duty nurses must be able to justify their actions as well as their decisions, which is not possible unless the nurse has the necessary knowledge.

Legal accountability applies to every citizen, and nurses like all other professionals are personally accountable through law for their actions or omissions. Such individual legal accountability is channelled through the criminal and civil law in the courts (Tingle 2004). The NMC 2008 code also emphasises that the nurse 'must act lawfully, whether those laws relate to professional practice or personal life'; thus accountability is continuous.

Litigation within healthcare in the United Kingdom has increased over the years and has huge financial implications for the NHS (Dougherty 2003). During 2006–2007 the NHS Litigation Authority (NHSLA) dealt with 5426 clinical negligence claims which cost £579.3 million. Over 80% of these cases were settled out of court (NHSLA 2008). The challenges of nursing within an increasingly complex healthcare framework, and the many competing priorities, mean that the risk of litigation is always present.

DUTY OF CARE
All nurses owe the patients they care for a duty of care. Liability is likely if that duty has been breached, the breach being a failure to meet the required standard of care. The standard of care required is determined by the Bolam test: 'the standard of the ordinary skilled man exercising and professing to have that special skill. A man need not possess the highest expert skill at the risk of being found negligent. ... it is sufficient if he exercise the ordinary skill of an ordinary man exercising that particular art' (*Bolam* v. *Fern Hospital Management Committee* 1957). This standard is well established as is *Bolitho* (1997): 'when challenged, if expert opinion could not withstand logical analysis then the judge has the right to conclude that the body of opinion is not reasonable or responsible' (Foster 2002). Consequently, when justifying clinical decisions or actions the practitioner would be expected to have considered their competencies within a particular situation as well as best practice principles if they were subject to litigation.

For a successful litigation the plaintiff must establish three principles on the balance of probabilities. These are:

- that a duty of care was owed by the defendant to the plaintiff
- that there has been a breach of that duty
- that, as a result of that breach, the plaintiff has suffered harm of a kind recognised in law and which is not too remote.

For example, a litigation claim could be evoked if in the course of her duty, a nurse inserted a peripheral cannula using poor technique which caused the patient an injury.

VICARIOUS LIABILITY

NHS Trusts and other employers have two forms of liability: (1) direct liability, i.e. the Trust itself is at fault; and (2) vicarious or indirect liability, i.e. the Trust is responsible for the faults of others, mainly its employees (Dimond 2005). It is a necessary requirement that the employee was acting within the course of their employment and that they were authorised to perform the procedure. For example, a nurse whilst caring for a patient obtains a blood sample from the patient and during the procedure the patient sustains a nerve injury. If the nurse did not have the necessary training or authorisation to perform the procedure, the patient would be able to claim clinical negligence. It is possible that the employer could seek to recover from the employee any compensation which may be paid out. However, the Department of Health advise against such practice (Dimond 2005).

The changing culture of clinical negligence claims has been reflected in the updated code of conduct. The NMC states that the nurse should have personal indemnity insurance and that if the nurse cannot arrange it then she must declare it to the person for whom she is caring as they need to be aware of that fact due to the potential for a clinical negligence claim. Such a declaration relates to registered nurses and not to non-registered healthcare personnel. Indemnity insurance is provided through professional organisations and trade unions.

RECORD KEEPING

Maintaining accurate records is fundamental to nursing practice and yet it is often overlooked, especially when workload demands are high. However, the NMC describes good record keeping as a 'tool for professional practice and one that should help the care process. It is not separate from this process and it is not an optional extra to be fitted in if circumstances allow' (NMC 2009).

Failure to document interventions accurately could have serious consequences. In terms of cannulation, records should demonstrate site selection, number of attempts and any problems encountered during the procedure. The record should be signed and dated with the time of insertion. Furthermore, records should demonstrate the care of the peripheral device as well as the outcome of treatment (Dougherty 2008). The nurse should remember that these records will be used in the event of a negligence claim being brought against her and will serve to protect her if the documentation is detailed and relevant. In the absence of relevant records, nursing practice can be called into question since there is no evidence to prove that the interventions took place. The nurse may also find it difficult to recall details since memory fades with time and recall can be scanty. Opinions may then be made about the nurse's fitness to practise because of failures in documentation, since 'good record keeping is an integral part of nursing and midwifery practice, and is essential for to the provision of safe and effective care' (NMC 2009). Furthermore, the practitioner and employer lose protection against negligence claims in the absence of clear and accurate records. Documents provided as evidence in court would be scrutinised and any failures would compromise the practitioner when they came to give evidence. Consequently, to neglect this area of practice is to open oneself to potential professional and legal complications.

CONSENT TO TREATMENT

The notion of consent is based on the principle of respect for the person and thus on the concept of human rights of life and liberty (Tschudin 2003). Central to the thinking about the nursing care of the patient is the philosophical concept of autonomy. On the premise that people know what is in their best interest, the ethical principle states that the choices of mature people must be respected and, reflecting this principle, the law insists that consent is, in the vast majority of cases, a prerequisite to the care of the patient (Cox 2001). As a registered nurse it is imperative that consent is obtained before any treatment or care is initiated. For consent to be valid the practitioner must ensure that consent is:

- given by a legally competent person
- given voluntarily
- informed (which includes information about the procedure as well as any known risks related to the intervention) (NMC 2008)

Consent may be given in a variety of ways and the law does not require consent to be given in a particular way. Implied, verbal, written and expressed consent are all equally valid; however, they can vary in their value as evidence in proving that consent was given (Dimond 2005). Examples of consent are: (1) a nurse is about to obtain a blood pressure reading and the patient holds out their arm for the procedure, then the consent is implied; (2) the nurse asks the patient if she can obtain a blood sample and the patient agrees, then the consent is verbal; (3) the nurse, prior to insertion of a central venous access device and following a comprehensive explanation of the procedure, asks the patient to sign a written document to confirm consent to the procedure.

Giving full explanations of what is being done, and why, how and when, is essential for the patient to remain a free agent and exercise the right to say no (Tschudin 2003). It is often difficult for nurses to accept a patient's refusal to give consent. However, an action of battery may be brought if treatment is given in the face of an explicit refusal of consent (McHale 2001).

EVIDENCE-BASED PRACTICE

The radical modernisation of the healthcare system that culminated in the publication of the NHS Plan (Department of Health 2000) empowered nurses to undertake a wide range of complex clinical skills which were traditionally the remit of the medical profession. The nursing profession has embraced the role expansion. However, the role expansion is inextricably linked with the risk of professional and legal complications for the nurse. The procedure of venepuncture and cannulation is commonly practised by nurses (Dougherty 2008). The importance of being competent to perform these procedures must never be underestimated since the consequences of bad technique and lack of knowledge can be serious. Skill is required to learn techniques and use equipment but of equal importance is the knowledge that is required to apply evidence-based practice, assess the patient, problem-solve, manage complications. A good knowledge of equipment is necessary to protect the practitioner from risks such as sharps injury, and agencies such as the National Patient Safety Agency (2007) advocate the use of needle-free systems whenever possible.

The NMC code (NMC 2008) states that each nurse must ensure that their practice is up to date; the notion of lifelong learning is inherent in the code and nurses are encouraged to actively seek out and comply with training programmes which will help inform their professional practice. Failure to maintain knowledge would be viewed as a breach of the code since the NMC emphasises the importance of maintaining competency in order to deliver safe and effective nursing care.

There is currently no national agreed training programme for venepuncture or cannulation; however, the RCN (2010) have published the third edition of their *Standards for Infusion Therapy*, which is essential reading for nurses performing venepuncture and cannulation. There is a risk in assumptions being made about the fact that such procedures, being commonplace, are easy to perform and require minimal knowledge. The reality is that in order for the nurse to deliver safe and effective care and to be competent to work without supervision she must demonstrate that she has maintained her knowledge and skill (NMC 2008).

It has become common practice for organisations to allow non-registered staff to perform cannulation and venepuncture following a period of training. If the procedure is being performed under the delegation of the registered nurse then she must be satisfied that the delegation is appropriate and be aware of the outcomes of the delegation. The nurse or midwife must:

- establish that anyone they delegate to is able to carry out their instructions
- confirm that the outcome of any delegated task meets the requires standards
- make sure that everyone they are responsible for is supervised and supported NMC (2008).

Clearly, the nurse is ultimately accountable for her actions as well as decisions.

CONCLUSION

The dynamic nature of healthcare makes it essential for nurses to keep up to date with advances in clinical practice to ensure they are fit for purpose. To ensure safe, effective and professional practice requires the nurse to maintain a good knowledge of the professional and legal requirements which influence the delivery of care.

REFERENCES

Clark, J. (2000) *Accountability in Nursing, Second WHO Ministerial Conference on Nursing and Midwifery in Europe*. Munich, 15–17 June 2000.

Cox, C. (2001) *The Legal Challenges Facing Nurses*. Discussion paper. Royal College of Nursing, London.

Department of Health (2000) *The NHS Plan: a plan for investment, a plan for reform*, Cm 4818-I. Department of Health, London.

Dimond, B. (2005) *Legal Aspects of Nursing*, 4th edn. Pearson Education, Harlow.

Dougherty, L. (2003) The expert witness. Working within the legal system of the United Kingdom. *Journal of Vascular Access Devices*, 8(2), 29–35.

Dougherty, L. (2008) Obtaining peripheral venous access. In: *Intravenous Therapy in Nursing Practice* (eds L. Dougherty & J. Lamb), pp. 225–270. Blackwell Publishing, Oxford.

Foster, C. (2002) Negligence: the legal perspective. In: *Nursing Law and Ethics* (eds J. Tingle & A. Cribb), pp. 75–89. Blackwell Science, Oxford.

Hodgson, J. (2002) The legal dimension: legal system and method. In: *Nursing Law and Ethics* (eds J. Tingle & A. Cribb), pp. 3–18. Blackwell Science, Oxford.

Hyde, L. (2008) Legal and professional aspects of intravenous therapy. In: *Intravenous Therapy in Nursing Practice* (eds L. Dougherty & J. Lamb), pp. 3–22. Blackwell Publishing, Oxford.

McHale, J. (2001) Consent to treatment I: general principles. In: *Law and Nursing* (eds J. McHale & J. Tingle), 2nd edn, pp. 89–109. Butterworth-Heinemann, Oxford.

National Patient Safety Agency (2007) *Promoting Safer Use of Injectable Medicines*. NPSA, London.

NHS Litigation Authority (2008) www.nhsla.co.uk (accessed 3 April 2008).

NMC (2008) *The Code. Standards of Conduct, Performance and Ethics for Nurses and Midwives*. Nursing and Midwifery Council, London.

NMC (2009) *Record Keeping: Guidance for Nurses and Midwives*. Nursing and Midwifery Council, London.

RCN (2010) *Standards for Infusion Therapy*, 3rd edn. Royal College of Nursing, London.

Tingle, J. (2004) The legal accountability of the nurse. In: *Accountability in Nursing and Midwifery* (eds S. Tilley & R. Watson), 2nd edn, pp. 47–63. Blackwell Science, Oxford.

Tschudin, V. (2003) *Ethics in Nursing. The Caring Relationship*, 3rd edn. Butterworth-Heinemann, Oxford.

Watson, R. (2004) Accountability and clinical governance. In: *Accountability in Nursing and Midwifery* (eds S. Tilley & R. Watson), 2nd edn, pp. 38–46. Blackwell Science, Oxford.

2 The Learning Experience

Sarah Phillips

LEARNING OUTCOMES

The practitioner will be able to:

❏ Evaluate if it is appropriate to learn these skills.
❏ Evaluate potential learning and assessment resources.
❏ Identify local learning opportunities.
❏ Realistically assess the complexities of learning within his/her own workplace.
❏ Consider his/her own and other professionals' needs when learning.
❏ Plan a successful route to achieve competency.

INTRODUCTION

This chapter explores different approaches to education, training and assessment for venepuncture and cannulation. As courses differ locally, strengths and weaknesses of educational methods are highlighted so that learners can avoid common pitfalls and identify potential resources. Competence is a theme throughout but has been specifically related to assessment approaches. The environment of work and learning is discussed, drawing on behavioural sciences to offer illumination on the complexities involved in learning at work. Different professional groups are later introduced so the learner can consider specific educational requirements for themselves and those around them.

Venepuncture and Cannulation, first edition. Edited by Sarah Phillips,
Mary Collins and Lisa Dougherty. Published 2011 by Blackwell Publishing Ltd.
© 2011 Blackwell Publishing Ltd.

Learners will benefit from taking time to consider if it is realistic and appropriate to acquire these skills in terms of gaining competency and maintaining expertise once competent. Training, education and development is only effective if what is being taught is needed and wanted and the reason for poor current uptake understood. Mager (1992) suggests these fall into two simple rules:

Rule 1: Training is appropriate only when two conditions are present:
- There is something that one or more people do not know how to do.
- They need to be able to do it.

Rule 2: If they already know how, more training won't help.

KNOWLEDGEABLE AND PRACTICAL LEARNING

Theoretical learning

The clinical area is rich with stimulating learning experiences but this can also be challenging for learners because it is also distracting. Learners therefore benefit from protected time in an environment conducive to acquiring theoretical knowledge including anatomy, physiology, specialised terminology and equipment design. An environment which has been designed for learning encourages active questioning because it should feel safer and less exposing for learners. Equally, patients need not experience discussions that may be anxiety-provoking and irrelevant to their own situation. This falls in line with the Essence of Care Benchmark for Communication. 'Communication takes place at a time and in a communication environment that is acceptable to all parties' (DH 2003b, p. 3).

Any division of theory and skill must be done carefully because it creates an artificial split that does not reflect the reality of healthcare roles, which require thinking and doing together. Benner *et al.* (1998) informs us that expert nurses make decisions about care by 'Thinking-in-Action' which is particularly relevant for these practical skills. Theory remains essential to provide a solid foundation to enable safe practice, but should not be the sole source of knowledge and understanding. Indeed it is too limiting for these skills because normal patient variation creates unpredictable outcomes that need to be learnt in practice. Mastering these skills therefore requires the learner to source learning tools and methods that are designed to include key theoretical elements (see Table 2.1) but also have a fundamental objective of facilitating integration of practical skill with theory.

Table 2.1 Key theoretical knowledge required

Anatomy:
- Anatomy and physiology of the normal arm including skin, veins, arteries and nerves and the feel and appearance of healthy veins including the presence of valves and junctions.
- Selection of vein and problems associated with venous access due to thrombosed, sclerosed inflamed and fragile veins, the effect on veins of ageing and the disease process, previous treatment, lymphoedema or the presence of infection.

Equipment:
- Improving venous access.
- Selection of device and other equipment.
- Appropriate collection tubes and precautions required.
- Components of the equipment and how the design can be optimised in practice.
- Risk management (reducing risk of needlestick injury, etc.).
- Performing the procedure (demonstration, techniques, etc.).

Patient:
- Assessment of patient needs.
- Importance of patient's identification and correct labelling and transport of specimens.
- Pharmacological and non-pharmacological interventions. (i.e., use of local anaesthetic or psychological management of anxious patients).
- Consideration of anatomical and physiological complications (injury, bruising, phlebitis).
- Infection prevention issues (hand washing, use of gloves, skin preparation, and waste disposal).
- Prevention and management of complications during insertion (haematoma, nerve injury, infiltration, extravasation, etc.).
- Monitoring and care of site (phlebitis assessments, flushing, dressing, removal of device).
- Patient information and education (leaflets, advice to notify staff of any adverse reactions).
- Professional and legal aspects (consent, professional guidance, knowledge and skills maintenance and documentation).
- Understanding of the rationale for the blood test or cannula.

Experiential learning

The diverse approaches to learning, including cognitive, social and humanist, offer useful sources to aid understanding of different responses to learning. According to experts from such disciplines, learning from experience is highly effective (Bion 1961; Gagné 1965; Knowles 1973, Bandura 1977; Rogers 1983). This is particularly positive for these skills because the clinical environment has an abundance of expertise and situations which naturally facilitate learning through experience.

Rogers (1983) believes that experiential learning has five qualities:

- It involves the whole person – both feelings and cognitive processes.
- It is self-initiated, with a sense of discovery coming from within.
- It is pervasive and makes a difference in the behaviour, attitudes and maybe the personality of the learner.
- It is evaluated by the learner, who knows if his or her needs have been met or not.
- The essence of it has meaning.

The lecture format is highly effective for some elements of the subject (as described above) but is lacking as a sole method of education for these skills. In fact, words could be viewed as inadequate for the task of trying to communicate distinct and minute patient and anatomical variations that will eventually make the difference between expert and novice practitioner. A combined practical and cognitive approach provides the optimal approach to effective learning and is readily available in clinical practice. Supervised practice, for example, utilises the rehearsal type of learning that Gagné (1965) informs us helps individuals to retain information for longer. In this way, the predominant psychomotor activities necessary for these skills require learners to organise responses, initiate the activity, monitor the process, and refine it with corrective moves after the first tries. Further, social learning is readily available, which Bandura (1977) reveals as advantageous because of the value of observing experienced role models. Finally, transferability is also increased as a result of students being able to practise knowledge and skills in a functional context, so that it is easier to imagine what it is like on the job (Bridges 1992).

Experiential learning, however, is fraught with difficulties for the learner, supervisor and organisation and this should be given some consideration before setting out to learn these skills. It is, in fact, logistically difficult to release two practitioners while ensuring work is completed. In addition to supervisors not always being available, practitioners have to take on the role of learner in front of colleagues and patients. Alternative and varied methods to achieve learning from experience should therefore be adopted to reduce these pressures. Experience does not have to be with patients and many things may be better learnt before facing usual patient variables. Mannequins, for example, allow the learner to master the equipment without alarming or causing discomfort to patients. Similarly, vein palpation can be learnt on colleagues and enables the learner to experience the value of touch when selecting the best veins. For detailed requirements for acquiring the practical elements of these skills see Table 2.2.

A combined approach of theory and practice

Procedures should be carried out by skilled practitioners, in such a way that the patient's anxiety and discomfort are minimised, complications are avoided and good venous access is preserved. Unskilled learners must therefore be guided and supervised so that a positive experience is achieved for patient and learner. A structured learning approach that incorporates appropriate knowledge acquisition with frequent and supportive practice will help the learner achieve a positive outcome such as those shown in Table 2.3.

Likewise in view of mounting service pressures in clinical environments there is a greater demand but reduced ability for staff to attend courses. The key to a high quality, knowledgeable healthcare worker therefore is not only theory but also guided, self-directed and supervised practical training (Collins *et al.* 2006). Knowles (1973) contends that adults prefer self-direction. Tools should therefore be practically based with clear guidance for the learner and assessor while adaptable for assessment of relevant knowledge according to specialty. The Vascular Access

Table 2.2 Key practical knowledge/skills required

The practitioner should be TAUGHT the skills in order to be able to:
- Assess the condition of a patient's veins, distinguish different structures and recognise and locate veins suitable for venepuncture or cannulation.
- Access suitable veins and achieve a successful outcome.
- Recognise and manage any complications arising during the procedure.
- Assess the patient's understanding of the procedure and give clear and understandable information at an appropriate level for the patient.

The practitioner should be SUPERVISED and assessed by someone who possesses the following:
- Clinical expertise in venepuncture and/or cannulation and be practising these skills on a regular basis.
- Have undertaken a teaching and assessing course or be an authorised assessor by the organisation as a suitable trainer.

In order to learn the PRACTICAL elements of the skill the practitioner requires the following:
- A simulation mannequin for initial practice (i.e., arm, hand or skin and vein).
- A suitable supervisor and/or assessor (see above).
- A range of blood sampling and cannulation equipment (safety devices wherever possible).
- Hand washing facilities.
- Appropriate skin cleansing equipment.
- Protective clothing (e.g. well-fitting gloves).
- Suitable means to improve venous access (e.g. tourniquets).
- Suitable equipment for safe disposal of sharps and dealing with blood spillage.
- Adequate facilities for staff and patient comfort (e.g. suitable chairs, cubicles, lighting, and temperature).

Professional practice
The practitioner will be educated and supervised in order to be able to:

Assess
- the physical and psychological status of the patient
- the patient's knowledge and consent to the procedure
- the appropriate equipment required to undertake the procedure successfully according to the patient's condition and venous access.

Perform
- the procedure according to organisation policy, a competency assessment tool and practice within the appropriate professional code of conduct.

Support
- the patient throughout the procedure through information giving and comfort measures.

Recognise
- when difficulties arise and manage where appropriate.

Acknowledge
- limitation and refer to more experienced colleague after a maximum of two failed attempts at the procedure.

Table 2.3 Outcome of a good learning experience

The patient considers that:
- She/he was made aware that the practitioner is learning a new skill and was able to raise any concerns without feeling pressurised to continue.
- She/he was given reassurance that the procedure would be performed safely and understands the role of the competent supervisor.
- She/he experienced as minimal physical and psychological discomfort as possible.
- She/he was treated as an individual.
- She/he was given the opportunity to ask questions throughout.
- She/he was able to stop the procedure at any point.
- She/he was taught the reasons for the procedure and the care of the site after completion.

The practitioner considers that:
- She/he held the patient's trust in his/her ability to proceed as necessary.
- She/he acquired necessary theoretical knowledge and was able to gain basic practical skills prior to clinical practice (i.e. using simulation equipment).
- She/he was able to gain access to practical support in the clinical environment.
- She/he had opportunity to practise in adequate amounts to build up skills and confidence.
- She/he had access to the learning resources listed above and equipment in the clinical area.
- She/he was able to gain assessment of both knowledge and skills from a competent colleague.
- She/he used a reflective practice process to guide future learning needs.
- She/he was able to practise within their professional code of conduct or organisation's policy.
- She/he is able to ask questions about technique.
- She/he can apply appropriate knowledge for the prevention and management of complications.

Network Structured Learning Programme (VAN 2008) assesses the learner's theoretical knowledge and practical skill(s). The level of expertise of the professional is assessed using a pathway (see Appendix Fig. 2.1 at the end of the chapter); the tool is adapted from Benner's (1984) novice to expert continuum (Appendix Fig. 2.2). The learner assesses her/himself initially, and then progresses from their self-assessed level of ability through to competency achievement. Learners self-assess each practice attempt and verify them with a supervisor (Appendix Fig. 2.3), complete questions relevant to the skill(s), include a piece of reflective work and take a final Objective Structured Clinical Examination (OSCE) (Appendix Fig. 2.4), which has assessor guidance (Appendix Fig. 2.5). This way of assembling and reviewing evidence of personal achievements is supported by Brown (1992) and Castledine (1994), who describe a portfolio as a 'dynamic positive means' to show that a person is demonstrating developing professional knowledge and competence. Personal and professional development are assessed in terms of: knowledge acquisition, psychomotor and interpersonal skills, academic and research skills, professional attitudes and behaviours.

LEARNING METHODS

Core knowledge can be found from a variety of sources. The learner may have options of formal study day(s), one-to-one training with an expert and self-directed study programmes either printed or technological. Organisations will differ in the structures and support they offer to achieve a positive learning experience (see Table 2.3) but whichever approach they adopt, their education programme must include certain aspects (see Table 2.1 and 2.2). There will also be organisation- and specialty-specific content that should alert the learner to national and local organisation gaps in current practice.

Formal study day

These are structured so the learner is clear about learning outcomes and how they will be achieved from the outset. The core theory is usually supplemented with some element of practice on a low-fidelity simulator, such as a mannequin arm or skin and vein. Learners will benefit by having fewer distractions compared to their working environment plus they will have protected time to learn. At the time of writing there are no nationally certified courses or comprehensive assessment processes for these skills; therefore a certificate only verifies attendance.

Common pitfalls

- Knowledge and skill are artificially split so have to be transferred back to the clinical environment.

- Release from clinical commitment is required and can result in late cancellation.
- Funding is required for staff replacement and course fees.
- Practical exposure is limited to artificial scenarios and equipment.

Simulation training

Low-fidelity simulation such as arms, skin and veins are relatively economical and effective for learning psychomotor skills and manipulation of equipment, angle of insertion and process of procedure. High-fidelity simulation includes computerised analysis of technique but is more expensive. Simulation equipment does not replicate the human situation or the variable clinical environment; it does, however, enable experiential learning in a safe environment; an approach supported by Cioffi (2001). Simulation has also been encouraged in the Institute of Medicine's 1999 report *To Err is Human: Building a Safer Health System* (Kohn *et al.* 1999, p. 179). Low-fidelity mannequins have been shown to be effective for some particular psychomotor skills (Stratton *et al.* 1991; Roberts *et al.* 1997). However, simulation needs to be used cautiously: Guillaume *et al.*'s (2006) research reveals simulation is effective in nursing education but has only proved beneficial when used appropriately and in a way that improves the quality of teaching and learning.

Common pitfalls

- Inappropriate use if guidance is not provided initially.
- Poorly maintained equipment.
- Simulated skin and veins do not replicate the real situation, making precision of insertion more difficult to master.

Self-directed study

Self-directed study offers a practical approach for learning while working because it can be completed at a time that suits the learner and at their own pace. It can also be done at a convenient time for the organisation and reduces logistical dilemmas associated with important clinical commitments.

Common pitfalls

- Lack of commitment from the organisation to give time back to the learner.
- Motivation to complete training in a reasonable timeframe.
- The necessary level of expertise or challenge from experienced others is difficult to incorporate effectively.

E-learning

Kruse (2004) advises that e-learning offers an individualised approach not possible from print media or instructor led courses: 'Like no other training form, e-learning promises to provide a single experience that accommodates the three distinct learning styles of auditory learners, visual learners, and kinaesthetic learners' (Kruse 2004, p. 1). Interactivity means that it is engaging rather than didactic and is therefore well placed for learning the troubleshooting techniques required for these practical skills.

Common pitfalls

- It is not as portable as a printed workbook, despite increased availability of hardware such as palmtop computers.
- It relies on technology which can be problematic and time-consuming.
- It adds a learning step for learners not proficient in computing.

Printed programmes

Printed programmes can be taken directly to the environment so that optimum learning is achieved because supervisor guidance is readily available. Theory can be studied at a pace that suits the learner and as all learning is documented supervisors can review learner progression.

Common pitfalls

- Paper documents risk being out of date by the time they are in print.

- Can be bulky and badly presented if there is a limited budget.
- Can get lost or damaged when completed in clinical environments.

Expert one-to-one training
Individual training and supervision by a practitioner who is expert in these skills is highly recommended if underpinned by adequate theoretical study. It encourages problem-based learning and can be learner led according to individual needs or speciality. Also, such real-world contexts and consequences not only allow learning to become more profound and durable, but increase the transferability of skills and knowledge from the classroom to work (Gallagher *et al*. 1992).

Common pitfalls

- It is reliant on the expertise of one individual, which is therefore limited to their experience and specialist background.
- The approach may be ad hoc because expert practitioners will have many priorities to balance.
- Costly to deliver.
- Limited availability.

ASSESSING LEARNING

Effective and necessary assessment
The need and effectiveness of clinical assessment is debatable especially when considering the inherent flaws of assessment processes. Limitations are created by the application of specific criteria to multiple individuals in order to ensure fair, reliable and accurate assessment. Also rigid tools may be detrimental to the professional, which Benner (1984) argues results in the definition of practice being reduced to the capabilities of measurement tools. Accurate appraisal from assessment is, however, identified as useful by Burns (1992). Nicklin & Kenworthy (1995) outline the benefits of assessment:

- Predict future behaviour.
- Measure achievement.
- Assess competence.

- Monitor students' progress.
- Motivate students.

Exactly what assessments measure is important yet problematic in clinical practice, and this is compounded further because determining competence is difficult; While (1994) points out that in general, notions of competence are often confused and misconstrued. The NMC offers some clarity: 'a bringing together of general attributes – knowledge, skills and attitudes. Skill without knowledge, understanding and the appropriate attitude does not equate with competent practice' (NMC 2008b, p. 3).

Assessments therefore become helpful in determining competence because they provide clearly stated criteria that enable the learner to demonstrate 'adequate ability, knowledge or authority' (Swannell 2003, p. 4). Professional bodies expand upon such simplistic definitions to clarify what is meant by competence for practice: 'You must have the knowledge and skills for safe and effective practice when working without direct supervision' (NMC 2008a, p. 4). It is closely related to scope of professional practice and encourages practitioners to be aware of their limitations: 'You must recognise and work within the limits of your competence' (NMC 2008a, p. 4). The Health Professions Council echoes this: 'You must act within the limits of your knowledge, skills and experience and, if necessary, refer the matter to another professional' (HPC 2008, p. 11).

Theoretical assessment

Theoretical assessment can be achieved effectively in a number of ways. E-learning-based assessments provide different questions each time and so ensure reliability, validity and fairness. Written assessments have the advantage of learners being able to expand on answers, they can be completed in any location and documentation can later be produced to demonstrate core knowledge as required (i.e. when changing role or following a clinical incident). The Structured Learning Programme (VAN 2008) offers an example of a written document that is intended to be reviewed with an assessor. In this way core knowledge is assessed and so assured, but questions can still be raised that may hold particular significance for patient group, previous learner experience or local and national issues.

Self-assessment and reflective practice

Marteau *et al.* (1989) and Crunden (1991) highlight difficulties of self-assessment in clinical practice. Learners may not always be able to accurately self-appraise competence because a poor outcome may be the result of a normal patient variation rather than technique. In the case of venepuncture and cannulation, for example, a learner may consider the procedure a failure if they do not access the vein. In contrast, an experienced supervisor may know the cause to be unavoidable and therefore assess the learner's overall approach as successful.

Reasons to adopt

- Self-assessment and reflection is recommended by regulatory bodies such as the Nursing Midwifery Council (NMC), General Medical Council (GMC) and Health Professionals Council (HPC). The GMC states: 'Graduates must be able to reflect on their practice, be self-critical and carry out an audit of their own work' (GMC 2003, p. 14).
- Modified self-assessment tools optimise adult learning approaches while remaining open to drawing on experienced others, a method endorsed by Dannefer *et al.* (2005). Runciman *et al.* (1998) also highlight that irrespective of the subjective nature of intuitive judgement, the expert opinion has much to offer.

Summative/final examination

National ratification of an assessment framework of these skills is not currently available in the United Kingdom. Indeed formal final assessments similar to models such as ALS (Advanced Life Support) which certify competence by successful completion, would not be realistic for such highly used skills.

Instead, final assessments tools that are locally endorsed could offer a more robust and accessible way forward. All assessments should be designed to demonstrate knowledge, skill and competency achievement and be sufficiently clear in order to avoid the need for retraining when changing roles. Comprehensive assessment guidelines are equally important in order to achieve a valid, reliable and fair assessment.

Reasons to adopt

- Acknowledges that learning has been achieved to specific standards. This gives clarity and a goal for the learner while assuring the organisation that a set level of competence has been achieved. It also provides clear evidence to professional bodies in the event of adverse clinical incidents.
- The Objective Structured Clinical Examination (OSCE) is an effective (final) assessment tool commonly used by medical schools in their clinical competence exams and is usually performed in a simulated environment or a skills laboratory (Reed 1992; Bramble 1994; O'Neill & McCall 1996).
- It is a clear and concise tool.
- The OCSE in its original simulated environment is argued as inadequate as a sole method of assessment for nursing students because it does not accurately replicate a ward environment (Cudmore 1997). However, adaptations to the OSCE to make it applicable in the clinical environment yet still objective have been made by the VAN (2008) (Appendix Fig. 2.5) and were reported as successful by Collins *et al.* (2006).

PROFESSIONALS LEARNING

Adult learner

Lorge (1947), writing about effective methods in adult education, suggested that to reach the adult learner, you have to teach what adults want. He stated that adults have 'wants' in the following four areas:

1. To gain something.
2. To be something.
3. To do something.
4. To save something.

Multi-professional learning

In the late 1990s in many hospitals junior doctors had responsibility for cannulation, although Dougherty (1996) reported that specialist nurses in the fields of cancer, cardiac and intensive care also fulfilled this role. Currently it is carried out by a range of suitably prepared healthcare professionals including, but not exclusively, nurses, paramedics, radiographers and healthcare support workers. The government and professionals endorse training and competence over a role-specific approach: 'Intravenous cannula insertion will be carried out by trained and competent staff using strictly aseptic techniques' (DH 2003a). It is suggested that cannulations are less traumatic when carried out by someone who has regular practice (Weinstein 2007; While 1994). Lavery (2003) also highlighted that frequent practice in enhanced clinical skills is essential. The decision as to who should practise venepuncture and/or cannulation should therefore be based on whoever is best placed to learn, maintain and update their skills. It should not be determined by professional status, prior experience or enthusiasm.

Each professional group will bring to these skills relevant experience according to their background and 'primary task' (Rice 1963, 1965). The primary task of a doctor, for instance, could be identified as diagnosing, compared to a nurse's primary task of caring. This understanding is useful when trying to understand puzzling responses or feelings of anxiety that can block competency achievement for these skills. Nurses, for example, must initially shift their role focus from 'caring' to 'curative', which may feel strange because it is at odds with their primary task. Likewise, a radiographer may feel challenged by doing more invasive procedures when compared to their regular diagnostic primary task. It is important that professionals are able to take time to integrate these skills into their practice in a way that works best with their own primary task.

Similarly, it is important for learners to appreciate the value of their own approach as well as those of other professionals, as the patient's experience may be equally positive. For example: 'a surgeon whose technical ability is critically important to his/her role' (Royal College of Surgeons 1999, p. 10) will have become an expert in the intricate psychomotor aspects involved in cannula placement. Initially this could be considered by the patient as favourable when compared to a carer with less developed psychomotor skills. However, in light of Boore's (1978) findings that anxiety can produce a similar physiological response as acute pain, the intensively developed communication skills of a carer may be of equal value to the patient. In this way, while the approach may vary, the level of pain and confidence experienced by the patient may be similar.

Post- and pre-registration learners

Nurses

Pre-registration nurse training does not normally cover venepuncture and cannulation within the curriculum, necessitating the need for post-registration training. A standardised pre-registration programme would help improve the practice of these skills and has been explored by the NHS in Scotland (NES 2004). Training may be incorporated into pre-registration training in the future, a concept which has previously been discussed for intravenous therapy (Ingram & Lavery 2005). Currently students should confirm the policy with their educational institution and placement organisation. They particularly need to ensure that it is appropriate for their stage of development and placement specialty and that they have the expected training and assessment required for these skills.

Post-registration nurses must follow professional guidelines and local policy if acquiring or refreshing their skills: 'You must take part in appropriate learning and practice activities that maintain and develop your competence and performance' (NMC 2008a, p. 4).

Allied healthcare professionals (AHP)

At times it will be appropriate for an AHP to be trained prior to registration (e.g. paramedics and operating department practitioners) because these skills form an integral part of their work. Therefore, AHP students who wish to learn the skills must first determine that it is a requirement for their role following registration and then check with the education and placement institution to ensure they are adhering to local policy and guidelines.

Registered AHPs currently number fifteen different professions (HPC 2011). Additionally as each role requirement varies according to type of work to be undertaken following qualification, a standardised approach to introduce venepuncture and cannulation into pre-registration curriculum would be inappropriate. Post-registration allied health professions have comprehensive standards as a guide to the best route for education, training and recording continuing professional development courses (HPC 2006).

Doctors

Pre-registration medical education in the UK has been radically reshaped in the past 15 years, prompted by the General Medical Council who drove, supported and monitored the changes since the first publication of *Tomorrow's Doctors* in 1993 (GMC 1993). Central aims of the reform included a reduction in curricular factual content and greater prominence of skills acquisition. The competency requirements explicitly outlined for doctors (GMC 2003) and the fact that medical students from some colleges are going though a structured learning approach (Collins *et al.* 2006) reflects a move away from the 'watch one try one' approach (Parker 1993). It is inappropriate for students to learn without support and it is the responsibility of registered doctors to ensure that students are properly supervised (GMC 2003). As other professions are practising these skills, supervision is more widely available, thereby reducing the pressure on medical staff. Indeed, Collins *et al.* (2006) reported that by using a structured learning tool, access to supervision from phlebotomists and nurses was opened up to medical students.

Post-registration doctors are deemed competent in these clinical skills by virtue of passing their practical examinations and underpinning theoretical study. However, if it has not been possible to maintain skills or review current evidence, guidance and support should be sought. 'You must keep your knowledge and skills up to date throughout your working life. You should be familiar with relevant guidelines and developments that affect your work. You should regularly take part in educational activities that maintain and further develop your competence and performance' (GMC 2006, p. 12). Additionally, hospitals may have local policy that requires doctors to demonstrate their current level of competency in these skills.

Healthcare support workers (HSW)

Registered practitioners are bound by their code of professional conduct and are accountable for their actions (GMC, NMC and HPC). In contrast HSWs are not regulated by a professional body so the decision to delegate is made either by the nurse or midwife or by the employer and it is the decision-maker who is accountable for it (NMC 2008a). It is therefore the responsibility of the employer or professional deciding to delegate to ensure appropriate training, supervision and assessment (NMC 2008a).

Until the current debate on the regulation of support workers addresses their role, careful delegation and robust practice procedures will continue to be necessary. National Vocational Qualifications (NVQs) or training programmes of equivalent robustness offer a sound way forward for ensuring competent and safe practitioners. These training programmes and supporting policies are then able to be ratified and authorised for use by the appropriate authority within the organisation. This ensures that individuals are not left in isolation with decisions to delegate which may be deemed inappropriate in retrospect and so it is in the best interests of the patient, employee (the person delegating and the person being delegated to) and employer.

Registered practitioners/nurses delegating

The registered practitioner is bound by their professional code of conduct to ensure the welfare of patients under their care. The NMC Code (2008a, p. 3), for example, states that nurses must consider three important elements before delegation:

- You must establish that anyone you delegate to is able to carry out your instructions.
- You must confirm that the outcome of any delegated task meets required standards.
- You must make sure that everyone you are responsible for is supervised and supported.

This is important for the person delegating but may also be helpful for the unregistered member who could otherwise not understand why their practice is under question. Further, the registered professional is obliged to reflect upon their choice of delegating the following the procedure: The nurse or midwife delegating an aspect of care has a continuing responsibility to judge the appropriateness of the delegation (NMC 2008a, p. 2).

While the code provides some clear boundaries, in reality it remains difficult for the organisation and registered practitioner to be sure of the appropriateness of delegation because of differences in each situation. The NMC supplementary guidance sheet on delegation is helpful here: 'The decision to delegate should be judged against what could be reasonably expected from someone with their knowledge, skills and abilities when placed in those particular circumstances (NMC 2008b, p. 1). Equally, the employer has a responsibility as part of this decision: 'to protect the public and support safe practice' (NMC 2008b, p. 2). The non-registered learner should therefore look for positive signs of support from the organisation or delegator in terms of clear management structures and systems including: education programmes, incident reporting and fair management of incidents, practice audit as well as periodic review of role activities.

The unregistered practitioner responsibility
Ultimately, the best person to determine if they are able to do the skill is the individual performing it as they can identify that they feel confident and appropriately placed. NMC (2008b, p. 2) states: 'Healthcare can sometimes be unpredictable. It is important that the person, to whom an aspect of care is being delegated, understands their limitations and when not to proceed should the circumstances within which the task has been delegated change.'

CONCLUSION
Learning the skills of venepuncture and cannulation has been shown to be more complex than it first appears. The clinical working environment offers an ideal arena for learning practical skills because it is stimulating, has lots of opportunities to prac-

tise and has a variety of experienced supervisors. Paradoxically it is not always a realistic place to take up the role of learner or teacher/supervisor effectively. Therefore, a combined practical and theoretical approach is suggested as a realistic and effective way forward.

Enthusiasm to learn and improve practice is always to be applauded; however, as a professional, the decision to take up these skills should only be made after determining if it is feasible to both learn and maintain them. It is hoped that learners reading this chapter will be encouraged to think realistically, yet positively, about how best to learn these skills in their own particular environment. These are essential procedures for patients and by having more professionals available to perform them well, and question how they are currently performed; patient experience can be much improved. In turn, practitioners have much to gain in terms of work and personal satisfaction by mastering them.

REFERENCES

Bandura, A. (1977) *Social Learning Theory*. Prentice Hall, Upper Saddle River, NJ.

Benner P. (1984) *From Novice to Expert: Excellence and Power in Clinical Nursing Practice*. Addison-Wesley, Menlow Park, CA.

Benner, P., Hooper-Kyriakides, P. & Stannard, D. (1998) *Clinical Wisdom and Interventions in Critical Care: A Thinking in Action Approach*. WB Saunders, London.

Bion, W.R. (1961) *Experiences in Groups*, p. 89. Brunner-Routledge, Hove.

Boore, J. (1978) In: *Surgical Nursing* (1997) (eds C. Torrance & E. Serginson), 12 edn, p. 132. Baillière Tindall, London.

Bramble, K. (1994) Nurse practitioner education: enhancing performance through the use of objective structured clinical assessment. *Journal of Nursing Education*, **33**(2), 59–65.

Bridges, E.M. (1992) *Problem Based Learning for Administrators*. ERIC Clearinghouse on Educational Management (ERIC Document Reproduction Service No. ED 347 617), Eugene, OR.

Brown, R.A. (1992) *Portfolio Development and Profiling for Nurses*. Quay Publishing, Lancaster.

Burns, S. (1992) Grading practice. *Nursing Times*, **88**(1), 40–42.

Castledine, G. (1994) How to compile a personal professional profile. *British Journal of Nursing*, **3**(10), 521–522.

Cioffi, J. (2001) Clinical simulations: development and validation. *Nurse Education Today*, **21**(6), 477–486.

Collins, M., Phillips, S., Dougherty, L., de Verteuil, A. & Morris, W. (2006) A structured learning programme for venepuncture and cannulation. *Nursing Standard*, **20**(26), 34–40.

Crunden, E. (1991) An investigation into why qualified nurses inappropriately describe their own cardiopulmonary resuscitation skills, *Journal of Advanced Nursing*, **16**(5), 597–605.

Cudmore, J. (1997) *Assessment of nursing students*. Royal College of Nursing Edlines Newsletter. Spring.

Dannefer, E.F., Henson, L.C., Bierer, S.B., *et al.* (2005) Peer assessment of professional competence. *Medical Education*, **39**(7), 713–722.

Department of Health (DH) (2003a) *Winning Ways: Working Together to Reduce Healthcare Associated Infection in England*. DH, London.

Department of Health (DH) (2003b) *Essence of Care: Patient-focused Benchmarks for Clinical Governance*, p. 3. DH, London.

Dougherty, L. (1996) The benefits of an IV team in hospital practice. *Professional Nurse*, **11**(11), 761–763.

Gagné, R.M. (1965). *The Conditions of Learning*. Holt, Rinehart and Winston, New York.

Gallagher, S.A., Stepien, W.J. & Rosenthal, H. (1992) The effects of problem-based learning on problem solving. *Gifted Child Quarterly*, **36**(4), 195–200.

General Medical Council (1993) As cited in General Medical Council (2003) *Tomorrow's Doctors. Recommendations on Undergraduate Medical Education*, 2nd edn. GMC, London.

General Medical Council (2003) *Tomorrow's Doctors. Recommendations on Undergraduate Medical Education*, 2nd edn. GMC, London.

General Medical Council (2006) *Good Medical Practice*. GMC, London.

Guillaume, A., Hunt, B., Gordon, R. & Harwood, C. (2006) Effectiveness of intermediate-fidelity simulation training technology in undergraduate nursing education. *Journal of Advanced Nursing*, **54**(3), 359–369.

HPC – Health Professions Council (2006) *Your Guide to Our Standards for Continuing Professional Development*. HPC, London.

HPC (2011) *About Registration – Professions*, p. 1. At: http://www.hpc-uk.org/aboutregistration/professions/ Last accessed on 19th January 2011.

Ingram, P. & Lavery, I. (2005) Peripheral intravenous therapy: key risks and implications for practice. *Nursing Standard*, **19**(46), 55–64.

Knowles, M. (1973) *The Adult Learner: A Neglected Species*. Gulf Publishing Company, Houston, TX.

Kohn, L.T., Corrigan, J.M. & Donaldson, M.S. (1999) *To Err is Human: Building a Safer Health System*. National Academy Press, Washington, DC.

Kruse, K. (2004) *The Benefits and Drawbacks of e-Learning*, p. 1. At: http://www.e-learningguru.com/articles/art1_3.htm (accessed 3rd August 2009).

Lavery, I. (2003) Peripheral intravenous cannulation and patient consent. *Nursing Standard*, **17**(28), 40–42.

Lorge, I. (1947) *Effective Methods in Adult Education: Report of the Southern Regional Workshop for Agricultural Extension Specialists*. North Carolina State College, Raleigh, NC.

Mager, R.F. (1992) *What Every Manager Should Know about Training*. Lake Publishing Company, Belmont, CA.

Marteau, T.M., Johnston, M., Wynne, G. & Evans, T. (1989) Cognitive factors in the explanation of the mismatch between confidence and competence in performing basic life support. *Psychology and Health*, **3**, 173–182.

NES – NHS Education for Scotland (2004) *Transferring the Skills: A Quality Assurance Framework for Venepuncture, Cannulation and Intravenous Therapy*. At: http://www.nes.scot.nhs.uk/documents/publications/classa/ClinicalSkillsdraft121004.doc (accessed 29 May 2009).

Nicklin, P.J. & Kenworthy, N. (1995) *Teaching and Assessing in Nursing Practice*, 2nd edn. Baillière Tindall, London.

NMC (2008a) *The Code: Standards of Conduct, Performance and Ethics for Nurses and Midwives*, p. 3. NMC, London.

NMC (2008b) *Advice Sheet on Delegation*. At: http://www.nmc-uk.org/aFrameDisplay.aspx?DocumentID=4184 (accessed 27 April 2009).

O'Neill, A. & McCall, M. (1996) Objectively assessing nursing practices: a curricular development. *Nurse Education Today*, **16**(2), 121–126.

Parker, S. (1993) Trading places. *Nursing Times*, **89**(45), 42–43.

Reed, S. (1992) Canadian competence. *Nursing Times*, **88**(3), 57–59.

Rice, A.K. (1963) *The Enterprise and Its Environment*. Tavistock Publications, London.

Rice, A.K. (1965) *Learning for Leadership. Selections from Group Relations Reader*, p. 71. Tavistock Publications, London.

Roberts, I., Allsop, P., Dickinson, M., Curry, P., Eastwick-Field, P. & Eyre, G. (1997) Airway management training using the laryngeal mask airway: a comparison of two different training programmes. *Resuscitation*, **33**(3), 211–214.

Rogers, C.R. (1983) *Freedom to Learn for the 80's*. Merrill, Columbus, OH.

Royal College of Surgeons of England. (1999) *Surgical Competence: Challenges of Assessment in Training and Practice*, p. 10. RCSENG – Communications, London.

Runciman, P., Dewar, B. & Goulbourne, A. (1998) *Project 2000 in Scotland: Employers' Needs and the Skills of Newly Qualified Project 2000 Staff Nurses*. Queen Margaret College, Edinburgh.

Stratton, S.J., Kane, G., Gunter, C.S., *et al.* (1991) Prospective study of manikin-only versus manikin and human subject endotracheal intubation training of paramedics. *Annals of Emergency Medicine*, **20**(12), 1314–1318.

Swannell, J. (ed.) (2003) *The Little Oxford Dictionary*, 6th edn. Clarendon Press, Oxford.

VAN (Vascular Access Network) (2008). *Structured Learning Programme for Venepuncture and Cannulation*, 2nd edn. Vascular Access Network, London.

Weinstein, S.M. (ed.) (2007) *Plumer's Principles and Practice of Intravenous Therapy*, 7th edn. JB Lippincott, Philadelphia.

While, A. (1994) Competence versus performance: which is more important? *Journal of Advanced Nursing*, **20**(3), 525–531.

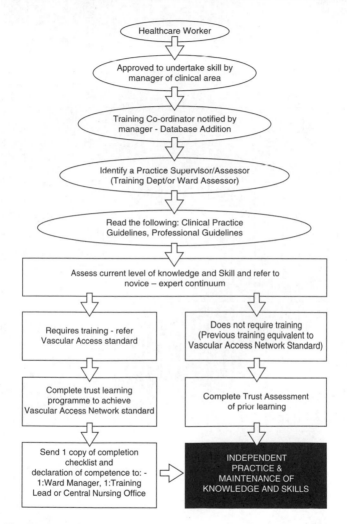

Fig. 2.1 Learning pathway for venepuncture and cannulation. With permission from Vascular Access Network.

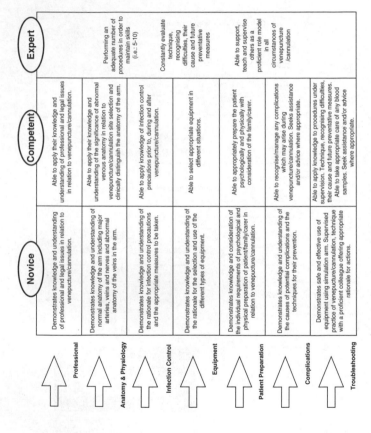

Fig. 2.2 Novice to expert continuum. With permission from Vascular Access Network.

Supervised Practice Assessments - Venepuncture

Self-Assessment, demonstrating competency progression under supervision

Name	
Job Title	
Organisation	
Department	
Clinical Skill	Venepuncture	Date started:		Date completed:	
Skill Supervisor's Name	1.		2.
Skill Supervisor's Name	3.		4.
Skill Supervisor's Name	5.

This form is a self assessment tool, but the practitioner will be able to discuss the rationale for each of the actions and demonstrate competency in the practical application of these skills as applicable

Skill Required	10 SELF ASSESSMENTS Achieved = Tick Not Achieved = 0									
	1	2	3	4	5	6	7	8	9	10
A. Correct identification of patient										
B. Appropriate patient preparation and communication										
C. Chooses and handles equipment confidently and correctly										
D. Considers personal safety and that of others										
E. Correct identification of suitable vein										
F. Appropriate venous dilation methods										
G. Provision of local anaesthesia as required (as per healthcare organisation)										
H. Needle inserted and sample obtained										
I. Correct order of draw for multiple samples										
J. Appropriate troubleshooting techniques										
K. Aseptic technique followed throughout										
L. Needle removed safely and care of site given										
M. Disposal of sharps safely										
N. Completes documentation, labelling, and sample dispatch (as per healthcare organisation)										
Initial of Skill Supervisor:										
Initial of Practitioner:										
Date:										

Fig. 2.3 Self-assessment. With permission from Vascular Access Network.

Final Assessment - OSCE (Objective Structured Clinical Examinations)

Essential skills, demonstrating competence for independent practice

Name	
Job Title	
Organisation	
Department	
Clinical Skill	Venepuncture
OSCE Assessor	
OSCE Question	Demonstrate the skill of Venepuncture
Date	

OSCE COMPONENT	Pass	Refer
1. Appropriate communication with patient throughout		
2. Demonstrates safe technique throughout the whole procedure		
3. Familiar with equipment		
4. Aseptic technique throughout		
5. Correct positioning of patient and preparation of environment		
6. Chooses appropriate vein and site for venepuncture		
7. Provides local anaesthesia (as per healthcare organisation)		
8. Completes venepuncture procedure correctly and safely (as per healthcare organisation policy)		
9. Disposes of sharps and equipment correctly and safely		
10. Completes documentation in line with local healthcare organisation		

Outcome	Pass		Refer	

OUTCOME AGREED			
Date	Practitioner	OSCE Assessor	
	Sign:	Sign:	
	Print:	Print:	

Fig. 2.4 Final assessment – OSCE (Objective Structured Clinical Examinations). With permission from Vascular Access Network.

COMPETENCIES	GUIDANCE
1. Appropriate communication with patient	Provides patient with full explanation of procedure. Obtains verbal consent from the patient for the procedure. Demonstrates caring and sensitive manner at all times. Employs methods to reduce patient anxiety.
2. Demonstrates safe technique throughout the whole procedure	Confirms patient identity against request form. Demonstrates safe practice to reduce risk of complications. Aware of personal safety and that of colleagues. Avoids causing damage to the vein. Bottles labelled at bedside once completed. Safe disposal of sharps. Aware of needle stick injury policy. Tourniquet not left on for too long (< 2 mins). Aware of local policy for number of attempts at procedure before referral to another colleague (normally two attempts). Considers risk associated with patient variants i.e.: Drug therapy (i.e. clotting) and disease processes.
3. Familiar with equipment	Demonstrates knowledge of different venepuncture equipment available. Considers patient's veins and indications for device before selecting appropriate equipment. Collects all equipment together before beginning procedure.
4. Aseptic technique throughout	Correct hand washing technique conducted before procedure. Checks packaging and dates of equipment to ensure sterility of equipment. Correct skin preparation. Maintains non-touch/aseptic technique during procedure.
5. Correct positioning of patient and preparation of environment	Assists patient into a comfortable position. Arranges lighting and self to ensure maximum effect. Addresses patient's concerns/requests appropriately.
6. Chooses appropriate vein and site for venepuncture	Demonstrates knowledge of anatomy and physiology of veins and related structures. Assesses veins visually and by palpation. Considers patient's individual physiological and psychological needs and able to state indication or contraindication for venepuncture site selection.
7. Provides local anaesthesia (as required)	Apply local anaesthetic if required, and ensures this is prescribed if necessary. Allows time for anaesthesia to take effect.
8. Completes venepuncture correctly and safely	Skin is cleaned according to local infection control policy and skin traction applied. Needle is inserted and stabilised with minimal discomfort to the patient. The correct volume of blood is obtained, in the appropriate bottle, in the correct order of draw. Tourniquets released, and needle removed with minimal discomfort. Digital pressure is applied to minimise bruising and bleeding. Universal precautions observed throughout, and sharps disposed of correctly. Bottles labelled at the patient bedside. Sample despatched correctly and timely. Demonstrates smooth psychomotor skills throughout.
9. Disposes of sharps and equipment correctly and safely	Sharps and equipment disposed of according to local healthcare organisation infection control policy.
10. Completes documentation in line with local policy	Documents venepuncture procedure/attempt or any problems, and labels bottles by the bedside and correctly (as per healthcare organisation).

Fig. 2.5 Assessment guidelines for venepuncture. With permission from Vascular Access Network.

3 | Anatomy and Physiology

Mary Collins

LEARNING OUTCOMES

The practitioner will be able to:

❑ Describe the parts of the circulatory system.
❑ Understand the anatomy and physiology of veins.
❑ Identify veins in the arm and hand.
❑ Explain the components of blood.

INTRODUCTION

The circulatory system consists of a network of blood vessels which transport blood and its components around the body. One type of blood vessel, namely veins, give access to the circulatory system. Veins do not, however, occur in isolation and therefore to avoid causing damage to arteries and nerves, anatomical knowledge is required to ensure adequate care is taken during the assessment and subsequent accessing of the vein for the procedures of venepuncture or cannulation.

OVERVIEW OF THE CIRCULATORY SYSTEM

The circulatory system consists of the pulmonary and the systemic systems. In relation to venepuncture and cannulation the systemic system, the larger of the two, is the most relevant for venepuncture and cannulation. It consists of the heart, functioning as a pump which requires a transport network that is made up of arteries, veins and capillaries to carry blood and its com-

Venepuncture and Cannulation, first edition. Edited by Sarah Phillips,
Mary Collins and Lisa Dougherty. Published 2011 by Blackwell Publishing Ltd.
© 2011 Blackwell Publishing Ltd.

ponents to and from the tissues (Herbert & Sheppard 2005; Weinstein 2007).

The heart is a muscular pump receiving deoxygenated blood from the body via veins that empty into its right chambers. These chambers are known as the right atrium and right ventricle (Marieb 2006). The blood on leaving the atrium and entering the ventricle is prevented from flowing back into the atrium by a valve (tricuspid). The heart pumps the deoxygenated blood out of the right ventricle, via the pulmonary artery to the lungs, where it receives oxygen and excretes carbon dioxide. The oxygenated blood returns to the left atrium and when the heart contracts the blood is forced into the left ventricle, where again a valve (mitral) prevents any backflow to the left atrium. The blood leaves the left ventricle in the aorta and it is carried around the body via arteries (Herbert & Sheppard 2005).

Blood flows around the heart and the body in a one-way system. In the heart the valves, e.g. tricuspid and mitral, control this one-way system (Marieb 2006). As oxygenated blood leaves the left side of the heart it is under immense pressure from the pumping action of the heart. This blood leaves the heart in the aorta and is taken around the body in arteries until it finally enters the capillaries. The capillaries connect to the veins and the deoxygenated blood is returned to the heart against gravity. The force of the pumping action of the heart is not present in the veins, and to facilitate the one-way system, veins contain valves that shunt the blood forward to enter the right side of the heart (Marieb 2006).

The blood transported in the veins has delivered its oxygen, nutrients and electrolytes to the cells and collects wastes for excretion (Marieb 2006). This is the specimen of blood obtained when venepuncture is performed and is the blood that fluids and medications are added too when a cannula is inserted into a vein.

ARTERIES, VEINS AND CAPILLARIES

The arterial system carries oxygenated blood to the tissues from the heart. This blood contains oxygen and it is therefore normally bright and cherry red in colour. The oxygenated blood leaves the heart in the aorta (which has a lumen of approximately 2.5 cm in diameter). The blood is under pressure from the contraction of the left ventricle and therefore the walls of arteries are thicker than veins (Marieb 2006). This pressure creates a pulse. The oxygenated blood is distributed around the body in arteries; each has a relatively large diameter of approximately 0.4 cm, which aids the blood flow. These arteries become smaller with each further branching and subdividing, most often referred to as arterioles, with a much smaller diameter of approximately 20 μm (Herbert & Sheppard 2005).

Capillaries are composed of endothelium, therefore are only one cell layer in diameter. This is why exchanges are easily made between the blood and the tissue cells, as the capillaries tend to form interweaving networks, called capillary beds (Marieb 2006). Blood in the capillaries is a mixture of arterial and venous blood, with arterial blood delivering oxygen, fluids and nutrients to the individual cells and venous blood collecting their carbon dioxide and wastes. Capillaries are sometimes referred to as exchange vessels. Capillaries have a diameter of approximately 6–8 μm, and it is estimated that there are 40000–50000 million in the body. The capillary network drains into a series of vessels that increase in diameter to form venules and veins (Herbert & Sheppard 2005).

The venous system acts as a collecting system, bringing blood from the capillaries back to the heart (Herbert & Sheppard 2005). This blood is low in oxygen (deoxygenated) and it is normally much darker and more bluish-red in colour than arterial blood. The walls of veins comprise the same three layers as the arteries but with less elastic muscle, therefore the walls of the veins are thinner than arteries. The lumen size of the venules and veins can be modified by contraction of the smooth muscle of the tunica media to alter the capacity of the venous system (Herbert & Sheppard 2005).

Approximately 60% of the blood volume is contained within the venous system (Herbert & Sheppard 2005). Maintenance of an adequate venous return to the heart is required at all times because the cardiac output depends on the venous return. The returning blood is flowing against gravity and some veins, especially in the arms and legs, have valves made up of folds of endothelium in the walls of the veins to prevent backflow

(Herbert & Sheppard 2005). Pooling of blood in the peripheral circulation is therefore prevented (Finlay 2004). The return of blood to the heart is primarily aided by two systems – the skeletal muscle pump and respiratory pump. Contraction of skeletal muscles, especially in the limbs, forces or squeezes the blood through the veins toward the heart due to the contraction and relaxation of the muscles surrounding the veins (Marieb 2006). The respiratory pump also assists the return of blood to the heart. When we inspire, the diaphragm contracts and increases the capacity for the thorax to allow the lungs to expand. This causes a decrease in the intrathoracic pressure which in turn causes the large veins near the heart, including the inferior vena cava, to expand and fill. On expiration the pressure changes but valves prevent backflow down the veins (Finlay 2004; Marieb 2006). Venous return is also aided by venomotor tone, which alters the capacity of the venous system by the modification of the lumen size, thus decreasing the capacity of the venous system.

STRUCTURE OF BLOOD VESSELS

Arteries and veins are composed of three main layers: tunica intima, tunica media and tunica externa (Marieb 2006). The thickness of each layer varies with the size and type of blood vessel (Fig. 3.1).

A cross-section of an artery or vein will reveal three layers of tissue (Fig. 3.1), known as tunics, each with a different function. The innermost layer, the tunica intima, which lines the lumen, is a thin layer of endothelium (squamous epithelial cells, one cell in diameter). The extreme smoothness of this layer prevents abnormal blood clotting but is prone to damage by the insertion of venous access devices, with trauma encouraging platelet adherence and thrombus formation (Finlay 2004; Weinstein 2007).

The following errors during venepuncture or cannula insertion will result in damage to the endothelial cells of the vein:

- inadequate skin preparation
- insertion of a cannula too large for lumen of the vein

- insufficient anchoring of the skin and vein during cannula advancement
- insertion of a cannula close to an area of joint flexion
- inadequate securement, allowing the cannula to move
- poor skin preparation and incorrect use of dressings, which can allow microorganisms to contaminate the site.
- inappropriate choice of vein that does not support infusion of fluids or medications (Hadaway 2001).

In veins, the tunica intima contains semilunar folds of endothelium called valves. Valves extend from the tunica intima into the lumen of the vein. They are found in most veins, most plentifully in the veins of the limbs, and function to keep blood moving towards the heart (Weinstein 2007). However, the exact location of valves within the superficial veins used for venepunc-

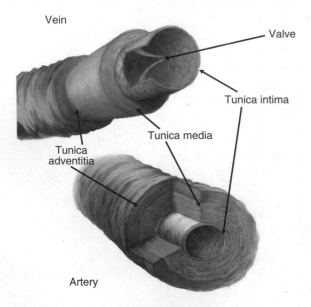

Fig. 3.1 Diagram of vein and artery. Used with permission of Becton, Dickinson and Company.

ture is not known due to the variation between individuals (Hadaway 2010). Valves are usually located in pairs and at points of branching and are present as a noticeable bulge externally in the vein (Hadaway 2010; Weinstein 2007). This bulge appears due to the distension of the vein when a tourniquet is applied (Hadaway 2010). When the suction is applied during venepuncture, the valves compress and close the lumen of the vein, preventing the flow of blood into the blood bottle (Weinstein 2007) or cannula advancement (Dougherty 2008) (see Chapter 9).

The tunica media or middle layer is made of smooth muscle that runs in rings around the vessel and elastic connective tissue. Veins have a thinner layer of smooth muscle than arteries and are more likely to collapse when pressure in the lumen is low (Weinstein 2007). The smooth muscle is stimulated by stretch. When it is overstretched, the muscles contract to resist that stretch. This is the physiological response when a tourniquet has been left in place longer than the recommended 2 minutes and the veins can no longer be palpated (Hadaway 2010).

Similarly, application of a tourniquet causes the smooth muscle fibres to elongate to contain the increased volume collecting in the veins. The pressure will increase quickly and then, within a few seconds, fall back toward the normal level, even with the increased volume. Removal of the tourniquet results in volume and pressure suddenly falling and within several minutes the normal pressure is re-established. This physiological process is important when removing a tourniquet and advancing a long cannula into a vein. Obstruction may be encountered if not enough time has elapsed to allow equilibrium to return (Hadaway 2010).

This middle layer is sensitive to changes in temperature, chemical or mechanical irritation, which can result in spasm of the affected vessel, and make insertion of the needle more difficult and painful at the site due to the change in blood flow (Finlay 2004; Weinstein 2007). Application of heat causes vasodilation, which will relieve the spasm, improve the blood flow and relieve the pain (Weinstein 2007) (see section in this chapter on the autonomic nervous system).

The tunica externa (or tunica adventitia) or the outer layer is a fibrous layer of connective tissue, collagen and nerve fibres. This layer is very strong, and therefore supports and protects the vessels. The vasa vasorum, a dense capillary network, supplies blood to the vessel walls. This network may penetrate to the tunica media in veins (Hadaway 2010).

THE NERVOUS SYSTEM

The nervous system controls the body's response to environmental changes using electrical impulses as a means of communication (Allan 2005; Marieb 2006). The nervous system is divided into the central nervous system and the peripheral nervous system. The peripheral nervous system relays the information to the central nervous system and most nerve impulses stimulating muscles to contract originate from the central nervous system (Marieb & Hoehn 2007).

Anatomical division of the central nervous system comprises the brain and the spinal cord, and the peripheral system includes all other nerve tissue that communicates between the brain and spinal cord. Twelve cranial nerves carry impulses to and from the brain and 31 pairs of spinal nerves carry impulses to and from the spinal cord (Marieb 2006; Weinstein 2007). The 31 pairs of spinal nerves are named according to the vertebrae where they emerge from the spinal cord: 8 cervical pairs, 12 thoracic pairs, 5 lumbar pairs, 5 sacral pairs and 1 very small coccygeal pair (Marieb 2006). Plexuses, which are complex networks of nerves, serve the motor and sensory needs of the limbs (Marieb 2006). The brachial plexus originating from C5–C8 and T1 contains the radial, median, musculocutaneous and ulnar nerves (Table 3.1).

The practitioner's knowledge of the proximity of these nerves to veins is important for venepuncture or cannulation as accidental puncture may cause damage to the nerves and the area of the body served by them (see Table 3.1). On the palm side of the hand the median nerve can be superficial, which may result in venepuncture being painful for the patient (Hadaway 2010).

The peripheral nervous system may be further subdivided into:

- somatic function
- autonomic function
- enteric function.

The somatic nervous system consists of sensory receptors – specialised structures located in various parts of the body that respond to certain stimuli in the environment, e.g. heat, light, pressure, pain or chemical (Weinstein 2007). The central nervous system is constantly informed of all events with messages transmitted along sensory or afferent nerve fibres to the central

Table 3.1 Brachial nerve plexus (Marieb 2006, with permission)

Plexus	Origin (from ventral rami)	Important nerves	Body areas served	Result of damage to plexus or its nerves
Brachial	C5–C8 and T1	Axillary	Deltoid muscle of shoulder	Paralysis and atrophy of deltoid muscle
		Radial	Triceps and extensor muscles of the forearm	Wrist drop – inability to extent hand at wrist
		Median	Flexor muscles of forearm and some muscles of hand	Decreased ability to flex and abduct hand and flex and abduct thumb and index finger – therefore, inability to pick up small objects
		Musculocutaneous	Flexor muscles of arm	Decreased ability to flex forearm or arm
		Ulnar	Wrist and many hand muscles	Clawhand – inability to spread fingers apart

nervous system (Marieb 2006). The motor or efferent nerve fibres transmit information in the opposite direction from the central nervous system to the spinal cord or to effectors (muscles and glands) through the spinal or cranial nerves and cause an effect on the body organs (Allan 2005; Tortora & Derrickson 2009).

The autonomic nervous system consists of the sensory receptors located in the internal organs, e.g. stomach and lungs responding to stimuli and informing the central nervous system and the motor nerve fibres transmitting nerve impulses from the central nervous system to the smooth muscle, cardiac muscle and glands (Tortora & Derrickson 2009).

Not all events are under voluntary control. The involuntary control is subdivided into two distinct parts: the sympathetic and parasympathetic nervous system (Allan 2005). The sympathetic nervous system innervates smooth muscle(the tunica media contains smooth muscle) and is associated with stressful situations, e.g. fear, pain, anxiety; the parasympathetic opposes the sympathetic effect and focuses on conservation of energy (Marieb & Hoehn 2007) and slowing of the heart rate and contractility. The sympathetic stimulation in a flight or fight situation, or if the vagus nerve in particular is stimulated, causes narrowing of the vessel known as vasoconstriction. This causes an increase in both heart rate and contractility, making venepuncture and cannulation difficult (Hadaway 2010). The vagus nerve innervates the heart. If it is provoked, for example by emotional stress, dehydration, and pain or prolonged standing, it will cause bradycardia and hypotension. This is known as a vasovagal reaction or vasovagal syncope (Weinstein 2007).

Reduced sympathetic stimulation will cause smooth muscle fibres to relax and the vessel lumen to increase, known as vasodilation. The patient who is relaxed will present less of a challenge for carrying out the procedures of venepuncture and cannulation.

LOCATION OF VEINS

Venepuncture and peripheral cannulation are performed in the veins that lie superficially to the epidermis, in the upper extremities of the body. They anastomose with one another and with

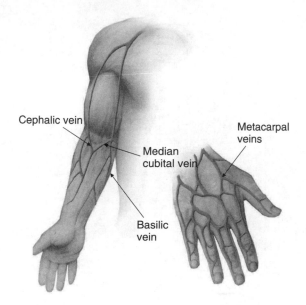

Fig. 3.2 Veins of the hand and arms. Used with permission of Becton, Dickinson and Company.

deep veins but they do not join arteries. Deep veins usually accompany arteries and have the same names as the corresponding arteries. As arteries, veins and nerves can be in similar locations (Fig. 3.2), care must be taken during the assessment and when performing the procedure to avoid arteries and nerves (see Chapter 5). The location of veins used for venepuncture and cannulation is presented in Table 3.2.

The digital veins flow along the lateral portion of the fingers but are small (Dougherty 2008). The digital veins unite to form the dorsal metacarpal veins and are easily visualised and palpated (Scales 2005). The superficial venous arch in the dorsum of the hand drains into the cephalic vein and basilic vein (Marieb & Hoehn 2007). The cephalic vein at this location is large enough for cannulation but irritation to the tunica intima can be caused by cannula movement as it enters the vein. Movement of the wrist may also cause discomfort for the patient. There are three

Table 3.2 Location of veins for venepuncture and cannulation (Weinstein 2007; Scales 2008)

Vein	Location	Advantages	Disadvantages
Digital	Lateral portions of the fingers	Ideal for short term use	Smaller than veins in forearm; in the older patient there is diminished skin turgor and loss of subcutaneous tissue. For cannulation, fingers may require splinting; may cause patient discomfort. Last resort for fluid
Metacarpal	Dorsum of hand.	Can be visualised and palpated easily; easily accessible	Needle insertion is painful due to increased nerve endings; wrist movement is decreased and site is at risk of phlebitis developing
Accessory cephalic	Runs along radial bone	Large vein, easily accessible; easily stabilised	Cannula may reduce patient's hand mobility if placed over point of flexion
Cephalic	Lateral aspect of the wrist, proximal to the thumb and antecubital fossa	Large vein; easy to stabilise	For cannula insertion at the wrist, may cause discomfort for the patient. During venepuncture slight movement of the thumb may cause the tendons (that control the motion of the thumb) to obscure the vein

Medial antebrachial	Runs along ulnar side of forearm	At the wrist end may be suitable for venepuncture	Is situated between two branches of median nerve. The proximity of site to nerve endings may cause pain and there is danger of infiltration at the site. Should be avoided if possible
Basilic	Posterior-medial aspect of the forearm	Large vein; easily palpated	May be difficult to access and observe. Needle penetrating the dermis and proximity to nerve endings may cause pain
Antecubital	Antecubital fossa: Median cephalic (radial side), median basilic (ulnar side); median cubital (in front of elbow joint)	Easy to stabilise; easily accessible	Variations in the medial veins may occur and careful evaluation and assessment of each patient is required for cannulation purposes. Valves occur at the junctions of the basilic and cephalic, causing obstruction during cannula advancement

long tendons that control movement of the thumb so slight movement of the thumb during venepuncture could easily obscure the vein (Hadaway 2010).

The basilic vein is usually a large vein, but may be overlooked due to its position on the posterior medial aspect of the forearm (Hadaway 2010). It can be easily palpated but accessing for venepuncture or cannulation may be difficult due to the angle required.

The median antebrachial veins ascend anteriorly in the forearms to join the basilic or medial cubital veins, sometimes both. As the median antebrachial ascends from the wrist the veins may appear suitable for venepuncture because they are usually situated between two branches of the median nerve; however, performing venepuncture at this site may be extremely painful (Hadaway 2010). The basilic and cephalic veins continue into the forearm.

The median cubital vein runs diagonally across the antecubital fossa connecting the basilic and the cephalic veins (Scales 2005). There is great variation in the pattern of veins in this area, with the median cubital vein not always visible (Dougherty & Lamb 2008). The basilic and cephalic and median cubital veins in the antecubital fossa are the most commonly used for venepuncture, due to prominence and visibility (Ellis 2006). Care must be taken with valves that may be located at the junctions of the following blood vessels: median basilic with basilic, median cephalic with basilic, and accessory cephalic and cephalic. These valves may prevent cannula advancement during cannulation (Hadaway 2010).

SYSTEMIC BLOOD FLOW

Blood flows in a closed system which is influenced by many complex interactions:

- composition of blood
- blood vessel diameter
- pressure within the vessels
- speed of blood flow
- changes that occur in response to the need to maintain homeostasis (Hadaway 2010; Tortora & Derrickson 2009).

If changes occur to blood flow then there is a reduced blood supply to meet tissue needs and when blood vessels are inadequately filled a condition known as circulatory shock occurs. The response of the body to these changes in systemic blood flow will make it difficult to identify veins for performing venepuncture and cannulation as intense vasoconstriction occurs. Maintaining an adequate blood flow to vital organs becomes a priority (Marieb & Hoehn 2007).

Composition of blood

Human blood appears as a homogeneous, opaque, somewhat syrupy fluid that is red in colour. Arterial blood is a brighter red colour and venous blood has a darker, dull red colour. A person has 4 to 6 litres of blood depending on their size. It has a pH range of 7.35 to 7.45 and is 3 to 5 times thicker than water. The general functions of blood are transportation, regulation and protection. It has both solid and liquid components. These include plasma, blood cells and platelets.

Plasma is a straw-coloured fluid and contains approximately 90% water. There are over 100 different substances dissolved in plasma, including electrolytes, hormones, plasma proteins, and various wastes and products of metabolism.

Plasma proteins: plasma contains between 60 g and 80 g of protein per litre. There are three major groups: albumin, fibrinogen and globulin.

Functions of the plasma proteins:

- intravascular osmotic effect
- contribution to the viscosity of plasma
- transport
- protein reserve
- clotting and fibrinolysis
- inflammatory response
- protection from infection
- maintenance of acid–base balance.

Cellular components of blood comprise approximately 45% of its volume. There are three major cell types: erythrocytes, leucocytes and thrombocytes.

Erythrocytes or red blood cells transport oxygen in the blood to all the cells of the body. Haemoglobin is the red-coloured protein pigment that transports the bulk of oxygen to the tissues. It also carries small amounts of carbon dioxide. In a healthy adult the range of red blood cells is 4.5–6 million/mm^3.

Leucocytes or white blood cells defend the body against damage by bacteria, viruses, parasites and tumour cells. Large variations in the number of leucocytes may occur in an individual from hour to hour as various physiological factors, such as exercise and emotion, cause white cells to enter or leave the circulation system. On average in a healthy adult the range of white blood cells is 4000–11 000/mm^3. White blood cells are less numerous than red blood cells and account for less than 1% of the total blood volume (Marieb 2006). There are five kinds of white blood cells which are classified into two groups: granular and agranular.

1. Granular leucocytes include neutrophils, eosinophils, basophils.
2. Agranular leucocytes include lymphocytes and monocytes.

Thrombocytes or platelets are necessary for haemostasis (prevention of blood loss). They respond quickly to a break in the blood vessel wall and initiate the clotting cascade to stop the blood loss from the damaged blood vessel wall. A normal platelet count for a healthy adult is 150000–300000/mm^3 (Marieb 2006). The blood should clot within 3–6 minutes. Placing a piece of gauze or applying pressure to the damaged area speeds up the clotting process, for example after venepuncture or on removal of cannula (Marieb 2006).

The clotting cascade involves three mechanisms:

- Vascular spasm: where the smooth muscle in the artery or vein contracts in response to the damage. Platelets in the damaged area release serotonin, which causes vasoconstriction, thereby making the diameter of the vessel smaller (Pocock & Richards 2006).
- Platelet plugs: when the endothelium is broken and the underlying collagen fibres exposed, the rough surface causes

platelets to become sticky and adhere to the edges of the break and to each other. The platelets form a mechanical barrier or wall to close off the break in the capillary and stem the flow of blood (Pocock & Richards 2006).

- Clotting: The stimulus for clotting is the break in the vessel, which causes a rough surface. The more damage there is, the faster clotting begins, usually within 15–120 seconds. However, if the platelet plug is not stabilised by fibrin fibres around the plug, it is likely to break down and bleeding will restart after about 20 minutes (Montague 2005). The chemicals involved normally circulate in the blood and include platelet factors, chemicals released by damaged tissues, calcium ions, and the plasma proteins prothrombin, fibrinogen, factor 8 and others synthesised by the liver (Pocock & Richards 2006).

Blood vessel diameter

The viscosity (thickness or stickiness) of blood is determined by two factors: the cells in blood (haematocrit) and the level of plasma proteins (Hadaway 2010; Tortora & Derrickson 2009). Viscosity is affected by vessel diameter. The centre of the larger blood vessels is where the most rapid flow is found, with the slower flow closest to the vessel intima (Hadaway 2010). Blood flowing through small vessels and capillaries has a higher viscosity. This is due to the velocity of flow decreasing due to their smaller diameter which will cause the viscosity to increase. Rouleaux, where the red blood cells adhere to each other and form a stack, can become lodged in constricted places within vessels (Hadaway 2010). Therefore inserting cannulae in vessels with small lumen will further decrease the velocity of flow, thus affecting the viscosity of blood. When choosing a cannula it is important to choose the smallest cannula for the largest vessel (Ortega *et al.* 2008). This will allow flow of blood between the cannula and the wall of the vessel. A knowledge of the patient's haematocrit (the erythrocytes, which normally constitute about 45% of the total volume of blood sample) and hydration status are therefore important (Hadaway 2010) to establish if velocity is affected, thus influencing the viscosity of blood and therefore choice of cannula.

Sympathetic nerves innervate the smooth muscle of all arteries and veins. This causes muscle contraction and vasoconstriction. Vasoconstriction is the term given when the muscle contracts the diameter of the vessel lumen and it becomes smaller (Herbert & Sheppard 2005). The rate of the sympathetic discharge is controlled by the cardiovascular centre in the medulla oblongata in the brain, known as the vasomotor centre. Increase in sympathetic discharge increases the venomotor tone, so the capacity of the venules and veins decreases and venous return increases. This control is very important in conditions such as haemorrhage (Herbert & Sheppard 2005).

Baroreceptors are nerve endings that influence the diameters of blood vessels. These nerve endings are located in the carotid sinuses and the aortic arch and are stimulated by the stretch of the blood vessel wall (Marieb & Hoehn 2007). Blood pressure produces this stretch and during haemorrhage when blood pressure is reduced, the baroreceptors are stimulated and send an impulse to the vasomotor centre to result in vasoconstriction, to increase the patient's blood pressure and allow venous return to increase and circulation to continue (Marieb 2006). Similarly, when a patient stands up having been sitting or lying down for a period of time and feels dizzy and light-headed due to the effect of gravity, vasoconstriction returns the patient's blood pressure to homeostatic levels (Marieb 2006).

The postganglionic sympathetic fibres normally release norepinephrine and this acts upon the smooth muscle to produce contraction and vasoconstriction. Epinephrine released from the adrenal medulla causes vasoconstriction in a similar way to the sympathetic nervous discharge. Nicotine also increases the release of epinephrine from the adrenal medulla and therefore causes vasoconstriction. Equally drugs that mimic the action of the sympathetic nervous system cause vasoconstriction, for example dopamine, epinephrine and norepinephrine (Herbert & Sheppard 2005).

Endothelium-mediated regulation

The endothelium, the innermost layer of blood vessels, can synthesise factors that can cause vasodilation, e.g. nitric oxide, and vasoconstriction, e.g. endothelin. A variety of agents (e.g.

acetylcholine, adenosine triphosphate, bradykinin, serotonin, histamine, shear stress of blood flow) can stimulate the endothelial cells to produce and release nitric oxide. Nitric oxide when released from the endothelium diffuses into the muscle layers surrounding the blood vessel walls. This makes the muscles relax and blood vessels dilate. It is this steady release of nitric oxide that keeps blood vessels dilated (Herbert & Sheppard 2005). Nitric oxide has also been found to inhibit platelet aggregation, an important phase in the natural haemostasis to stop blood loss when a blood vessel wall is damaged (Herbert & Sheppard 2005; Marieb & Hoehn 2007). Another important function of the endothelium is to prevent clot formation. Numerous factors that prohibit or promote coagulation are found in the endothelium, e.g. thrombomodulin, prostacyclin, tissue plasminogen activator, tissue factor pathway inhibitor and von Willebrand factor (Montague 2005). If these cells are damaged during cannulation, e.g. by too rapid advancement of the cannula, failure to correctly anchor the skin and vein, or inadequate skin cleansing (see list in 'Structure of blood vessels' section, above), then the inflammation process of phlebitis and thrombosis commences (Hadaway 2010).

Chemical control of blood vessel diameter

Chemical factors such as hormones and locally produced metabolites also affect the vascular smooth muscle. Angiotensin II, formed by the action of renin on angiotensinogen released in response to hypotension, causes vasoconstriction. Histamine and plasma kinins, released as part of the inflammatory response when tissues are damaged, cause vasodilation of the small vessels (Herbert & Sheppard 2005).

Response to local metabolites

Increasing blood flow in response to local demand is known as active hyperaemia. The precise nature of the metabolites that produce this relaxation of the smooth muscle (vasodilation) are not known (Herbert & Sheppard 2005). Many factors have been proposed as vasodilators, e.g. lack of oxygen, high levels of carbon dioxide and lactic acid, decreased pH, hyperosmolarity of the interstitial fluid, adenosine and prostaglandins.

If, for example, the tourniquet is left on a patient's arm for longer than 2 minutes, the blood supply to the arm is occluded for that time. While the occlusion remains the cells are metabolising, and the metabolites are accumulating, as there is no blood flow to remove them. Once the tourniquet is released blood flow is restored. This vasodilation has resulted in an enlarged capacity in the capillary system; therefore the arm is 'redder' in appearance than the other arm, known as reactive hyperaemia (Herbert & Sheppard 2005).

Circulatory shock will alter the normal physiology of blood vessels. Homeostasis is unbalanced and depending on the type of shock, fluid balance is interrupted. There is resistance to blood flow, due to increased capillary permeability and vasoconstriction of the peripheral blood vessels (Dougherty 2008). Access to peripheral veins when this occurs is very difficult and central access may be the most appropriate option.

Speed of blood flow
The velocity or speed of blood flow differs in the various blood vessels. The larger the diameter of the blood vessel, the slower the blood will flow. Blood is forced into large thick-walled elastic arteries that expand as the blood is pushed into them when the ventricles contract (Marieb 2006). This high pressure forces the blood to continually move into areas where the pressure is lower. The capillaries have the lowest pressure, with a blood speed of 0.3–0.5mm per second (700 times lower than in the aorta because of the diameter) (Herbert & Sheppard 2005). This allows the exchange of gases and nutrients to take place. This part of the circulatory system is often referred to as the microcirculation (Herbert & Sheppard 2005). Because the blood speed in other vessels is much quicker, this makes the circulation time quite short. The time it takes for the blood to go from the right ventricle to the lungs, and back to the heart to be pumped by the left ventricle to the body and return to the heart again is about 1 minute or less; this is known as the circulation time (Herbert & Sheppard 2005). As previously mentioned, the flow of blood is one way, and this is assisted by skeletal muscles relaxing and contracting and the 'respiratory pump'.

INTEGUMENTARY SYSTEM

The blood vessels are protected by the integumentary system or skin. The skin protects the entire body from damage that may be caused by chemicals, thermal or mechanical injury and bacteria. It has a rich network of capillaries and cutaneous sensory receptors. The skin is composed of two main layers: epidermis and dermis.

Epidermis

The epidermis, the superficial part of the skin, varies in thickness and is made of keratinised stratified squamous epithelium, which covers and protects the body. The keratinocytes are arranged in four or five layers known as strata that form the epidermis. Parts of the body that have exposure to friction, sunlight and abrasion will have five layers of keratinocytes (Tortora & Derrickson 2009). Manual labourers who for example have exposure to these elements may have veins that are more difficult to access for cannulation or venepuncture (Hadaway 2010).

The epidermis is avascular with no blood supply of its own. Cells on its surface are dead and continually flake off (Marieb 2006). Over 3 million microorganisms live on the epidermis. These microorganisms have adapted to the conditions of the skin and are known as resident or normal flora. They live in deep crevices in the skin, in hair follicles and sebaceous glands. The type and distribution of the organisms vary according to the body site, temperature, humidity and the person's general health. The largest number of microorganisms resident on the skin are Gram-positive bacteria, e.g. coagulase-negative staphylococci, micrococci and coryneforms (Wilson 2006).

The epidermis and the dermis are firmly connected; however, if interstitial fluid accumulates in the cavity between the layers, they will separate, e.g. blister, burn.

Dermis

The dermis is made of fibrous connective tissue and helps to hold the body together. The dermis varies in thickness like the epidermis and consists of two major parts – the papillary layer and the reticular layer (Marieb 2006).

The papillary layer lies immediately beneath the epidermis. It anchors the epidermis and contains small, finger-like projections called dermal papillae that indent the epidermis with some containing capillary loops that supply nutrients to the epidermis (Marieb 2006). Other dermal papillae contain sensory nerve endings, e.g. Meissner corpuscles, that are sensitive to touch. The cellular arrangement between these two layers prevents the epidermis shearing off the dermis when shearing forces are applied to the skin (Edwards 2005). The reticular layer is the deepest skin layer and contains blood vessels that play a role in maintenance of body temperature. As well as capillaries in the dermis, there are arterioles and the smooth muscle in their walls permits them to constrict and dilate. In a warm environment the arterioles dilate (vasodilation), allowing excess heat to be radiated to the environment. In a cold environment, the arterioles constrict (vasoconstriction) and heat is kept within the core of the body. Vasoconstriction can also occur during stressful situations. Blood flow to the dermis may be interrupted by prolonged pressure on the skin and without its blood supply the skin dies (Marieb 2006).

The skin is the largest sensory organ in the body and the dermis contains the rich nerve supply, which alert us to touch, pressure, pain and temperature changes (Edwards 2005). Neurons carry impulses from the cutaneous sensory receptors to the central nervous system. The skin contains three main types of sensory nerve endings: unspecialised free nerve endings, specialised nerve endings (or encapsulated) and specialised non-neuronal (or separate) receptor cells (Allan 2005; Tortora & Derrickson 2009). These sensory receptors function in response to a specific stimulus, e.g. mechanoreceptors, thermoreceptors, nociceptors, osmoreceptors and chemoreceptors (Tortora & Derrickson 2009). Chemoreceptors do not have a direct effect on the procedure of venepuncture and cannulation (Hadaway 2010). A variation of stimulation generates the free nerve endings, for example mechanical stimulus, such as the application of touch and pressure when palpating veins or application of tourniquet (Hadaway 2010). Ruffini's endings (a specialised nerve ending) respond to stretching when the digits or limbs are moved in preparation for the insertion of a needle during venepuncture or cannulation. Thermoreceptors are free nerve endings that sense warmth and cold. A cold environment will result in vasoconstriction and impede the flow of blood. A warm environment promotes vasodilation, improving blood flow in the blood vessels being accessed (Weinstein 2007). Free nerve endings(nociceptors) that occur throughout the skin are sensitive to painful stimuli (mechanical and chemical stimuli of varying intensity, extreme heat or cold, touch). These sensory receptors respond to stimuli arising outside the body and serve to protect the skin from injury in the environment and the information can be acted upon rapidly by the central nervous system (Edwards 2005). The nerve supply varies in different areas of the body. Some areas are highly sensitive, e.g. the inner aspect of the wrist, and other areas are only mildly sensitive. The insertion of a needle in one area may cause greater pain to the patient, yet in another patient it may cause minimal or no pain. This is why the inner aspect of the wrist is only used for venepuncture as a last resort (Weinstein 2007).

Ageing process
Veins deteriorate with age. The walls of the vein become weaker and stretch. The valves lose their competency and cause pooling of blood. This makes the veins more mobile, more fragile and often thrombosed and tortuous (Dougherty 2008). The dermis and epidermis become thinner and more fragile, and there is a reduction in subcutaneous tissue, resulting in less support for the blood vessel but making it easier to see veins clearly (Marieb 2006). The thickness of the epidermis varies with age; in an older patient, the skin on the dorsum of the hand may be so thin it does not adequately support the vein for venepuncture (Weinstein 2007).

CONCLUSION
Veins are a direct route into the circulatory system and to safely cannulate or perform venepuncture for patients, the healthcare practitioner must have a sound theoretical knowledge of the anatomy and physiology of blood vessels. Other considerations

for performing these two procedures include composition of blood, blood vessel diameter, blood flow, the skin and ageing process. Before accessing the vein, the healthcare practitioner must use this knowledge to assess the vein and reduce the risk of complications for the patient.

REFERENCES

Allan, D. (2005) Sensory receptors and sense organs. In: *Physiology for Nursing Practice* (eds S. Montague, R. Watson & R. Herbert), 3rd edn, pp. 133–148. Baillière Tindall, UK.

Dougherty, L. (2008) Obtaining peripheral venous access. In: *Intravenous Therapy in Nursing Practice* (eds L. Dougherty & J. Lamb), 2nd edn, pp. 225–270. Blackwell Publishing, Oxford.

Dougherty, L. & Lamb, J. (eds) (2008) *Intravenous Therapy in Nursing Practice*, 2nd edn, pp. 225–270. Blackwell Publishing, Oxford.

Edwards, S. L. (2005) Innate defences. In: *Physiology for Nursing Practice* (eds S. Montague, R. Watson & R.A. Herbert), 3rd edn, pp. 635–683. Baillière Tindall, UK.

Ellis, H. (2006) *Clinical Anatomy, a Revision and Applied Anatomy for Clinical Students*, 11th edn. Blackwell Publishing, Oxford.

Finlay, T. (2004) *Intravenous Therapy*. Blackwell Science, Oxford.

Hadaway, L.C. (2010) Anatomy and physiology related to infusion therapy. In: *Infusion Nursing: An evidence based approach* (eds M. Alexander, A. Corrigan, L. Gorski, J. Hankins & R. Perucca), 3nd edn, pp. 139–177. Saunders Elsevier, Philadelphia. (eds J. Hankins, R.A. Lonsway, C. Hedrick & M. Perdue), 2nd edn, pp. 65–97. WB Saunders, Philadelphia.

Herbert, R.A. & Sheppard, M. (2005) Cardiovascular function. In: *Physiology for Nursing Practice* (eds S. Montague, R. Watson & R. Herbert), 3rd edn, pp. 383–463. Baillière Tindall, UK.

Marieb, E. (2006) *Essentials of Human Anatomy and Physiology*, 8th edn. Pearson Benjamin Cummings. USA.

Marieb, E. & Hoehn, K. (2007) *Human Anatomy and Physiology*, 7th edn. Pearson International, USA.

Montague, S.E. (2005) The blood. In: *Physiology for Nursing Practice* (eds S. Montague, R. Watson & R. Herbert), 3rd edn, pp. 335–381. Baillière Tindall, UK.

Ortega, R., Sekhar, P. Song, M., Hansen, C.J. & Peterson, L (2008) Peripheral intravenous cannulation. *New England Journal of Medicine*, **359**(21), e26–29.

Pocock, G. & Richards, C.D. (2006) *Human Physiology, The Basis of Medicine*, 3rd edn, pp. 225–246. Oxford University Press, Oxford.

Scales, K. (2005) Vascular access: a guide to peripheral venous cannulation. *Nursing Standard*, **19**(49), 48–52.

Scales, K. (2008) Anatomy and physiology related to intravenous therapy. In: *Intravenous Therapy in Practice* (eds L. Dougherty & J. Lamb), 2nd edn, pp. 23–48. Blackwell Publishing, Oxford.

Tortora, G.J. & Derrickson, B. (2009) *Principles of Anatomy and Physiology*, 12th edn. John Wiley & Sons, Inc. USA.

Weinstein, S.M. (2007) *Plumer's Principles and Practice of Intravenous Therapy*, 8th edn. Lippincott Williams & Wilkins, Philadelphia.

Wilson, J. (2006) *Infection Control in Clinical Practice*, 3rd edn. Baillière Tindall, London.

4 Selection of Equipment

Mirjana Dojcinovska

LEARNING OUTCOMES

The practitioner will be able to:
- ❏ Identify the key components of the systems.
- ❏ Understand how to use the equipment correctly.
- ❏ Identify the different blood-collecting systems for venepuncture.
- ❏ Understand the significance of equipment design in achieving best and safe practice.
- ❏ Know how to select the most suitable device for each procedure.

INTRODUCTION

There are two aspects central to modern medicine: safety and accuracy. The long-term aim, including that of today's medicine, has consistently focused upon moving towards 'smarter' and more integrated developments. Therefore, if in previous centuries the aim was to obtain intravenous access, today the aim is towards more closed intravenous systems, where drugs and fluids enter the patient's veins but micro-organisms cannot and where patient and user safety and comfort are the paramount consideration (Rivera *et al.* 2005). Likewise; in the previous century, laboratories paid most attention to the analytic phase of testing, today the attention has shifted towards the pre-analytic phase in the collection of blood samples. Currently, most of the testing errors (32–75%) occur during the pre-analytic

Venepuncture and Cannulation, first edition. Edited by Sarah Phillips, Mary Collins and Lisa Dougherty. Published 2011 by Blackwell Publishing Ltd. © 2011 Blackwell Publishing Ltd.

phase, (Stankovic & Smith 2004), in comparison to analytical and post-analytic phases. This chapter aims to offer insight, knowledge and detail about the blood-collecting systems and their intended use so that practitioners will be fully informed about what equipment to use, and how and why they should use that equipment according to each situation.

VENEPUNCTURE

Needles and tubes

There are different sets of equipment for venepuncture. The choice will depend on the condition and the size of the patient's veins, required number of blood specimens, availability of the equipment and the practitioner's knowledge and skills. At present, blood can be drawn using:

1. vacuum tube system
2. winged blood collection set
3. syringe system
4. specialised equipment for neonates.

Vacuum tube system

The vacuum tube system (VTS, Fig. 4.1) is the most efficient method for obtaining a blood specimen (Garza & Becan-McBride

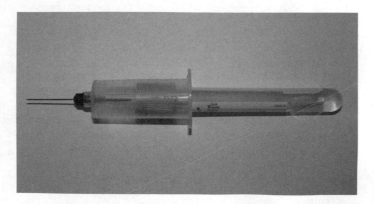

Fig. 4.1 Vacuum tube system (VTS). Used with permission of Vein Train Ltd.

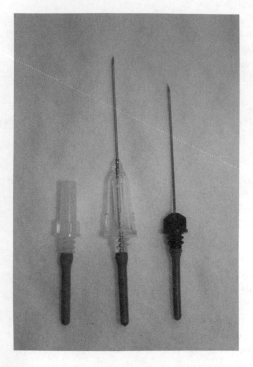

Fig. 4.2 Multi-sample needles including flashback needle. Used with permission of Vein Train Ltd.

2002; McCall & Tankersley 2008). It is a closed system in which the patient's blood flows through a needle inserted into a vein, directly into a vacuumed collecting tube without being exposed to the air. Though the designs of different manufacturers may vary, all VTS systems have three basic components:

1. multi-sampling double-ended needle (Fig. 4.2), or winged blood-collecting needle (Fig. 4.3)
2. transparent plastic holder to secure the needle and hold the vacuumed tube (Fig. 4.4)
3. vacuumed tubes (Fig. 4.5).

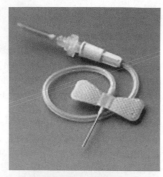

Fig. 4.3 Winged blood collection set with multi-sample needle pre-attached.

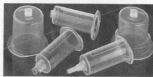

Fig. 4.4 Needle holder/bottle holder.

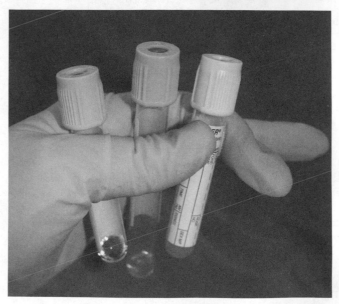

Fig. 4.5 Vacuum blood collection bottles. Used with permission of Vein Train Ltd.

Needles

Multi-sampling needle

All blood-collecting needles are sterile, disposable and designed for single use only. They are also silicone coated to help penetration through the skin and vein walls, and therefore less traumatic and less painful for the patient (McCall & Tankersley 2008). They are called multi-sampling because they allow multiple tubes of blood to be collected during a single venepuncture. In addition, some of the newest brands also allow flashback visualisation once the needle enters the vein (Fig. 4.6).

The VTS needle has two ends: a patient end, which is longer and bevelled for piercing the skin and entering the vein; and a non-patient end with rubber sleeve for penetrating the rubber top of a collecting tube. This rubber sleeve is retractable and is

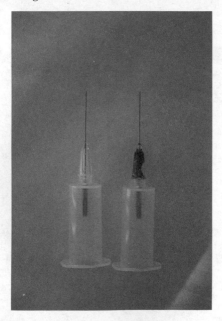

Fig. 4.6 Flashback needle demonstrating flashback. The needle on right shows example of flashback within the hub of the needle. Used with permission of Vein Train Ltd.

pushed back when the needle penetrates the rubber top of a tube, and recovers when the tube is removed, thus preventing blood leakage when changing the tubes during multiple tube draw. In the middle, the needle is threaded, separating the two different ends, and the threaded section is to enable the screwing of the needle into the needle holder.

Winged blood-collecting needle

The winged blood-collecting needle is a multi-sampling needle as well; the difference is that the two ends of the needle are separated by a permanently connected 12–30 cm length of tubing. In addition, at the point where the patient end of the needle joins the tubing there are plastic extensions that resemble butterfly wings, thus their popular name 'butterfly' (Fig. 4.3).

The winged blood-collecting sets are particularly useful for collecting blood from small or difficult veins. It allows more flexibility and precision than other needles, and has the advantage of visualisation of the flashback of blood as soon as the needle enters the vein. Though more expensive than any other device for venepuncture, they have become increasingly popular and in some centres they are the method of choice for venepuncture (Sommer *et al.* 2002).

Choosing the right needle

It is essential to match the size of the needle to the size of the vein (NCCLS 1991). When using large diameter needles, a large amount of blood enters the tube at once with great force, resulting in cell lysis. On the other hand, if needles are too small, red blood cells (RBCs) are forced to enter the needle through its small opening under great force, causing cell membrane shearing and release of the cellular components into the blood. The reliability of tests such as potassium, sodium, glucose, creatinine, bilirubin will then be decreased, resulting in falsely elevated test results (Stankovic & Smith 2004).

Gauge

The gauge system for sizing medical equipment is used widely around world. Yet, its origins and interpretation have long been obscure (Iserson 1987). The gauge, formally known as the Stubs Iron Wire Gauge, was developed in early nineteenth century in

England. Initially it was for use in wire manufacture, and each gauge size arbitrarily correlated to multiples of 0.0010 inches. This sizing system was the first wire gauge recognised as a standard by any country. In medicine, in the early twentieth century, it was used to measure needle sizes only. Today the International Organization for Standardization (ISO) also uses the gauge system to measure needles, catheters and sutures.

The gauge (G) number relates to the external diameter and is defined and regulated by ISO. The external diameter and the gauge number have an inverse relationship, that is, the larger the gauge number, the smaller the actual external diameter of a device.

For the needles, the gauge system is slightly complicated because for the same gauge there are two different inner diameters depending on the thickness of the walls (ISO 9626, 1991; ISO 9626, Amendment 1 2001).

Multi-sampling needles that are used for routine venepuncture are from 20G to 22G. For easy identification, manufacturers use a colour code for each gauge, and in general, they have colour-coded caps and hubs: for example, yellow for 20G, green for 21G and black for 22G.

For winged blood collection sets, the most commonly used are those of 21G and 23G. In rare situations, a 25G is used for collecting blood from tiny veins, or in neonates from the scalp. However, practitioners need to be aware that using a needle smaller than 23G increases the chances of causing haemolysis of the sample (McCall & Tankersley 2008).

Length

Needles also differ in their length; for venepuncture most are from 1.7 to 2.5 cm. Length selection depends primarily upon user preference and the depth of the vein.

Needle integrity

The needles come in a sterile packing: multi-sampling needles are enclosed in sealed twist-off shields or caps that cover both ends; butterfly needle are in sterile packs. It is important to examine the packaging or seal and expiry date before use. If the packaging is open or the seal is broken, or out of date, the needle is considered as no longer sterile and should not be used (see the Chapter 6). It is also important to visually inspect a needle before venepuncture. Needles are mass manufactured and on rare occasions contain defects, such as blunt or bent tips, or rough bevels or shafts that could injure a patient's vein, cause unnecessary pain, or result in multiple attempts to bleed the patient. If this happens, all needles from that brand should be withdrawn, as for any other faulty medical device, the Incident Reporting Form completed, and then submitted (by the supplier) to the Medical Device Agency for further investigation.

Holders

The second component of the VTS is the transparent plastic cylinder with a tube/bottle holder or needle holder (Fig. 4.4). It is an integral part of the system, making a firm, stable and safe connection between the tube and the multi-sampling needle. It has a small opening for screwing the needle into the top end. The other end is wide open to accept the collection tube and has two extensions to aid placement and removal of the tube.

Holders come in different sizes to fit tubes of different diameters: standard sizes that fit regular diameter tubes; smaller ones for small diameter tubes used in paediatrics, and the special large size for blood culture bottles (Fig. 4.7). These have an additional adapter to fit standard sized tubes (Fig. 4.7), which allows multiple blood collections after blood cultures specimens.

Some of the holders have an incorporated safety mechanism, such as a protective shield that manually locks the needle after it is withdrawn from the puncture site, e.g. BD Vacutainer System, Preanalytical Solutions (Fig. 4.8), or devices that manually or automatically retract the needle into the holder, e.g. Vanish point, Retractable Technologies, TX, by Greiner Labortechnik. For any of the holder safety devices, disposing of the holder while it is still attached to the needle ensures that the puncturing needle remains protected during and after disposal.

Vacuumed blood-collecting tubes

These colour-coded and vacuum-filled tubes are specifically designed for the task and are central to today's venepuncture (Fig. 4.5, Table 4.1). They are part of the vacuumed tube system and winged blood-collecting sets but can be used with a syringe system as well. They contain various additives, which are indicated by the colour of their cup or stopper (see Table 4.1).

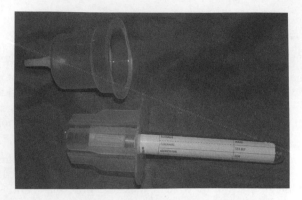

Fig. 4.7 Large bottle holder adaptor. Used with permission of Vein Train Ltd.

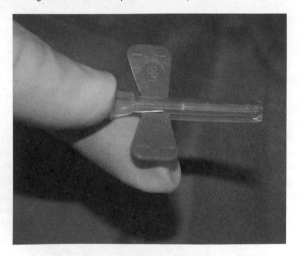

Fig. 4.8 Safety winged blood collection set. Used with permission of Becton Dickinson.

Vacuum

The vacuum system withdraws a premeasured and precise volume of blood. The practitioner should ensure the tube is filled to the mark indicated on the tube. Filling the right volume of blood is important in order to achieve the required blood to

Table 4.1 Vacuum Tube System Bottle choice – Order of Draw

Tube	Additive	Specimen	Determinations	Instructions
Blood Culture	Culture medium + Sodium Polyanethol Sulfonate (anticoagulant)	Whole blood	Aerobic followed by anaerobic – if insufficient blood for both culture bottles, use aerobic bottle only	
Light Blue	Sodium citrate	Plasma	PT, INR, APTT, TT, D-dimers, fibrinogen, thrombophilia screen (required 4 Sodium citrate tubes + 1 EDTA tube), Lupus (required 3 Sodium citrate tubes)	Tube must be completely filled. Gently invert 3–4 times
Red	No additive; silicone particles lining the tube's wall act as clot activator	Serum	IMST, B12, Antibiotic assays, Steroid hormones	Do not need inversions
Gold	Clot activator + gel for serum separation	Serum	For routine chemistry tests, Lipids, Thyroid (TFT), Drug levels (including lithium) , Proteins; NB- for Troponin I provide one separate tube	Gently invert 5–6 times
Green	Sodium heparin or Lithium heparin + gel for plasma separation	Plasma	For plasma determinations in chemistry	Gently invert 8–10 times
Lavender	EDTA	Whole blood	HBA1C, FBC, Reticulocytes, Sickle Screen, haemoglobin Electrophoresis, Red Cell Folate, Malaria, direct Coombes Test, Lead, Thalassaeima. Mercury, PTH, G6PD, ESR, IMST, Kleihauer	Gently invert 8–10 times
Pink	EDTA	Whole blood	Group and Antibody Screen. Have a special cross-match label	Gently invert 8–10 times
Grey	Sodium Fluoride + (K)oxalate	Plasma	Essential for Alcohoi, Glucose, Lactate	Gently invert 8–10 times
Royal Blue	Heparin or EDTA or none	Plasma or Serum	Trace elements- Zinc, Selenium, Manganese, Whole Blood	Gently invert 8–10 times

additive ratio, which is essential for some tests (CLSI, 2007 and CLSI 2008).

The Order of Draw

The order of draw refers to the sequence blood collection tubes should be filled. The needle that pierces the tubes can carry additives from one tube into the next. The order of draw makes sure that should cross contamination occur, it will occur with the least interference to the results.

The current order of draw according to CLSI (2007) standard H3-A6 is as follows. Practitioners should check their organisation's local policy for bottle choice and order of draw.

1.) Blood cultures SPS (sterile)
2.) Light blue (buffered sodium citrate tube)
3.) Red (plain), or Gold (gel separator tube)
4.) Green heparin and light green (sodium or lithium with or without separators)
5.) Lavender (EDTA)
6.) Pink, white
7.) Grey (Na fluoride/potassium oxalate)

The syringe system

The method of choice for blood sample collection is the vacuumed tube system. However, in patients with extremely difficult, fragile or small and collapsing veins a syringe system may be preferable, because a syringe can provide more controlled and gentle vacuum than the vacuumed tube.

Blood specimens collected with a syringe must be transferred to vacuumed tubes. The needle is simply pushed through the top of the tube, and blood is automatically be pulled into the tube because of the vacuum. This practice is unsafe with a high risk of needlestick injury so practitioners should not use syringe and needle without safety measures. A safe transfer can be achieved by using a safety transfer device which allows transfer of the blood without using the collection needle (Fig. 4.4). In addition, to ensure the quality of a specimen, the plunger of the syringe must not be pushed down when the tubes are being filled from the syringe, because it is extremely hazardous, as forceful expulsion can result in damage to the cellular components of the blood, which causes haemolysis (Stankovic & Smith 2004). If a safety transfer device is not available, then the venepuncture needle should be discarded into a sharp bin, then the vacuumed tube should be opened and blood decanted slowly down the side of the tube. Forceful injection of the blood to the bottom of the tube is hazardous and must be avoided. Also, samples need to be immediately transferred to an appropriate specimen tube to limit the clotting process that will be occurring inside the syringe (NCCLS 1991).

The syringes commonly used for venepuncture are 5 mL and 10 mL, depending on the size and condition of the patient's vein and the amount of blood to be collected. The larger syringes increase the likelihood of excessive aspiration pressures, blood clotting and haemolysis during collection and prior to transfer to a collection tube. Before using a syringe, the plunger needs to be loosened by withdrawing and pumping it 2–3 times (Sommer *et al.* 2002). There are safety syringes available with a shield that slides over the needle after use.

Needles for syringes

The needles used with syringe system are hypodermic, and they come in a wide range of sizes. The most common in use for venepuncture are those between 21G and 23G with a length of 2.5–3.7 cm.

Safety

The syringe and needle system for blood collection is regarded as a high risk procedure for splash and needlestick injuries. According to the EPINET Report in 2001, more than one-third of all needlestick injuries happened by using syringe and needle. In addition, the quality of specimens may be affected while transferring into the tubes. The rationale for using a syringe and needle system is very limited, therefore it should be avoided as much as possible.

CANNULATION

History

'Up to eighty percent of all patients admitted to hospital worldwide will receive a peripheral IV and this procedure is now considered indispensable to human health' (Rivera *et al.* 2007). The history of intravenous therapy is relevant to the current use of cannula development because it demonstrates the advances already made.

The first written document about intravenous therapy is from 1492 (Mainardi 1743): that resulted in death and accusations of murder. Almost two centuries later, in the early and mid 1600s, medical advances paved the way to a better understanding of anatomy and physiology. It was Christopher Wren who created the first working IV infusion devices, which he made from a feather quill and a pig's bladder (Corrigan 2001).

After fatal failures surrounding transfusion the Royal Society in 1668 banned all blood transfusions, followed by the Vatican and the French Government. (Corrigan 2001). It was only during the nineteenth century, disease, notably cholera, raised the importance of blood transfusions and IV therapy. The first infusions were administered: normal saline (Thomas Latta, 1832), glucose (Claude Bernard, 1843), and Ringer lactate (Sidney Ringer, 1876). In turn, the crude IV devices from the seventeenth century were replaced by metal needles, rubber tubing and glass containers. (Corrigan 2001).

Later, the plastic revolution in the 1950s changed medical practice as a whole, introducing disposable and single-use equipment. The first cannula was made in 1950. It looked very much like today's epidural needle and consisted of a shortened 16G needle with another steel needle as an inner stylet, and then over the top of the needle was fitted a polyvinyl chloride (PVC) catheter. The entire unit measured 5 cm and was available only in the 16G size (Massa 1951).

Components and design of the modern cannula

The components of today's cannula are shown in Fig. 4.9. Each of these components has a specific role, and they have been subjected to continuous developments – improving in their design and in material as well.

The *hypodermic needle* of the cannula is made of stainless steel, and it is silicone coated for easy sliding through the plastic cannula. The geometry of the needle tip is important for reducing pain during insertion.

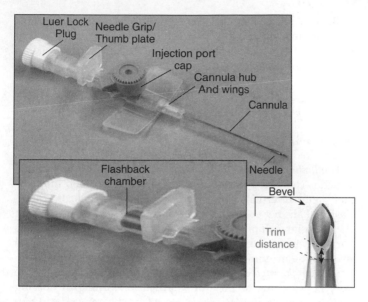

Fig. 4.9 Components of the cannula. Used with permission of Vein Train Ltd.

The *intravascular part of the cannula* – to which the term 'cannula' is applied, has changed the most, mainly due to the development of the plastics that constitute it. The first cannulae were made from polyvinyl chloride (PVC). PVC catheters were stiff, did not easily slide over the needle and into the vein, and were associated with a high rate of infusion phlebitis and bacterial adherence (Maki & Ringer 1991). Then, in 1969, TFE Teflon plastic was invented. The catheters made of Teflon were more flexible, more resistant to bacterial colonisation, self-lubricated and slid easily off the needle, and were non-compliant to pressure; Teflon proved to be non-toxic, tissue compatible but tough (Jacquot *et al.* 1989).

Further developments in the plastics industry brought a new plastic, polyurethane. The first polyurethane over-the-needle catheter was introduced in 1983. Polyurethane proved to be less traumatic to veins. Studies have shown that Vialon polyurethane catheters reduce the incidence of severe phlebitis by nearly 50%, in comparison to Teflon catheters (Maki & Ringer 1991); because of their flexibility they are less likely to kink and obstruct and therefore may also have a lower infection and thrombosis risk (Gaukroger *et al.* 1988; McKee *et al.* 1989). In addition, some types of polyurethane (e.g. PEU-Vialon, BD) are rigid at room temperature, but become more flexible after insertion, thus decreasing irritation to vein walls and reducing phlebitis (Stanley *et al.* 1992). In addition, due to the reduced risk of phlebitis, the optimum indwelling time for Vialon cannulae is longer, 3–4 days, in comparison with Teflon ones that need to be changed every 2 days (Maki & Ringer 1991).

The *flashback chamber* is a chamber at the back of the cannula which is connected to the needle and fills with blood immediately after insertion. The more rapid and reliable the blood flashback the better, as this prevents the needle from traversing the opposite wall of the vein (transfixation). Rapid flashback is currently provided by notched needles. Some experimental needles use magnifiers at the flashback chamber or hub.

Injection port and cap in ported cannulae – ported cannulae are very popular due to the port's structure assisting in holding and therefore easing IV access. However, they have disadvantages because of the high risk of infection from the port and also from blood spillage. During injection of medications, for instance, contact occurs between the unsterile syringe cone and the injection port. The repeated and unavoidable contact by hands of practitioners causes contamination, which due to product design cannot be decontaminated effectively. In fact studies showed that ported cannulae (Fig. 4.10) are associated with 55% bacterial contamination (Oberhammer 1980), and that the injection port acts as a sump, retaining a meniscus of fluid, which cannot be cleaned before or after the injection procedure. In addition, minute air emboli can been seen to enter via side ports at each injection and allow entry of bacteria (Pilsworth 1981).

An alternative to ported cannulae are *non-ported cannulae* (Fig. 4.11). They were designed with the aim of avoiding the risks associated with the ported cannula, and are used extensively in the USA and parts of Europe. IV access is achieved by adding extension tubing or the extension tube is an integrated part of the cannula (Fig. 4.12).

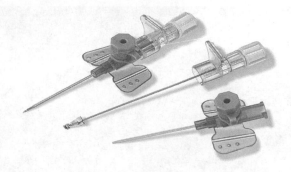

Fig. 4.10 Ported cannula (safety). Used with permission of B Braun Medical.

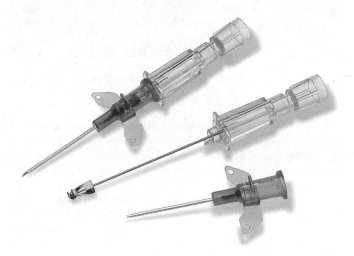

Fig. 4.11 Non-ported cannula (safety with wings). Used with permission of B Braun Medical.

The *wings* of the cannula have a supportive role during insertion, and help to secure the cannula in situ for the duration of use. It is made of transparent plastic to allow clear visibility of the puncture site (Rivera *et al.* 2005). This feature is important as it allows observation of the cannula and early detection of infection, phlebitis or bleeding around the cannula.

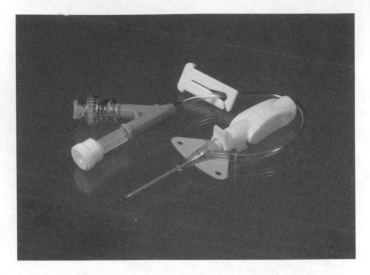

Fig. 4.12 Cannula with extension tubing incorporated. Used with permission of Becton Dickinson.

The *needle grip* also has a supportive role -to allow a good grip of the whole cannula before and during insertion, and allows the 'flicking' process (see Chapter 7) that helps to disconnect the Luer-lock plug from the needle at the moment of needle disposal into a sharps bin.

Multi-lumen port access can be provided by connecting an additional port on the cannula itself, by the attachment of a stop-cock or by using of an extension tubing (either attached or integral to the cannula) with multiple ports.

Choosing the right cannula

The size of a cannula

Gauge
Gauge is the external diameter of the intravascular part of a cannula and is regulated by the international standards (ISO 10555-5). Gauge size, abbreviated G, is denoted by a number; the smaller the number the larger the catheter. For example, an

Table 4.2 A guide to choosing the correct cannula

Colour	Gauge	Approximate flow rates (L/hour)			Comments
		Crystalloid	Plasma	Whole blood	
Orange	14G	16.2	13.5	10.3	Used in theatres or emergency for rapid transfusion of blood or viscous fluids
Grey	16G	10.8	9.4	7.1	Used in theatres or emergency for rapid transfusion of blood or viscous fluids
White	17G	7.5	6.5	4.6	Blood transfusions, rapid infusion of large volumes of viscous liquids
Green	18G	4.8	4.1	2.7	Blood transfusion, parenteral nutrition, stem cell harvesting and cell separation, large volumes of fluids
Pink	20G	3.2	2.9	1.9	Blood transfusion, large volumes of fluid
Blue	22G	1.9	1.7	1.1	Blood transfusions, most medications and fluids
Yellow	24G	0.8	0.7	0.5	Medications, short term infusions, fragile veins, children
Yellow (N)	24G	1.44			Neonatal

Adapted from Dougherty & Lamb (2008).

18-gauge catheter (18G) has a larger diameter than a 24-gauge one (24G). Each gauge size is identified by a standard colour, as required by ISO 10555-5; these are listed in Table 4.2.

Which gauge of the cannula to use will depend on the condition of a patient's veins, the type and amount of a infusate and the required speed of a infusion. A good cannula to vein ratio is

Good Cannula to Vein Ratio

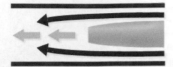

Poor Cannula to Vein Ratio

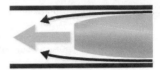

Fig. 4.13 Correct cannula to vein ratio.

Box 4.1 A good choice for cannula

A good cannula should provide:

- rapid, reliable blood flashback
- clear visibility of puncture site
- reduced pain to patient
- minimal injection risk
- minimal thrombotic risk
- dynamic softening of the catheter in the vein
- minimal blood exposure for the user
- multi-lumen port access
- needleless access to ports
- easy to apply a dressing to it.

---

important in order to secure adequate blood flow around the cannula (Fig. 4.13) and therefore to prevent phlebitis and obstruction of the cannula. A general guide is provided in Box 4.1.

Safer (needle) devices

The term 'safer needle devices' applies to all needles which have safety features (engineering controls) that prevent needlestick injuries. It is a broad term and includes many different types of devices, from those that have a protective shield over the needle to those that do not use needles at all. Based on mechanism of activation of safety features, safety devices can be categorised either as active or passive. Box 4.2 outlines the recommended safety features.

Passive safety features remain in effect before, during and after use; the practitioner does not have to activate them. Passive features enhance the safety design and are likely to have a greater impact on prevention. An example of such a product

---

Box 4.2   Safety features

Safety features designed to protect from needlestick injuries should:

- provide a barrier between the hands and needle after use
- allow or require the practitioner's hands to remain behind the needle at all times
- be an integral part of the devices and not an accessory
- be in effect before disassembly and remain in effect after disposal to protect downstream workers
- be simple and self-evident to operate and require little or no training to use effectively (UNISON 1999)

---

would be a spring-loaded retractable syringe or self-blunting blood-collecting devices (Figs 4.10 and 4.11).

Active devices require manual activation of the safety feature. An example of such a product would be needles with a sheath that must be manually pushed over the used needle (Fig. 4.8).

Safety for all our futures

Needlestick injuries and mucocutaneous exposure to infected body fluids can lead to considerable distress for healthcare practitioners, and to the transmission of bloodborne viruses. The viruses of major concern today are HIV, hepatitis B and hepatitis C. In an average hospital, workers incur approximately 12–30 needlestick injuries per 100 hospital beds each year (Eucomed 2008). However, it is estimated that between 60% and 80% of incidents go unreported. The Health Protection Agency (UK) reported that the number of percutaneous exposures to bloodborne viruses seen in medical professionals increased by 46% from 159 in 2002, to 232 in 2005. Following an injury from a contaminated 'sharp', the risk of transmission of infection is 1 in 3 for hepatitis B, 1 in 30 for hepatitis C and 1 in 300 for HIV (HPA 2006).

Needlestick and splashing injuries cannot be totally eliminated, but they must be combated at source. In the USA, in the 1990s, the Centers for Disease Control and Prevention (CDC) launched a multi-hospital study and showed that drawing blood is one of the highest-risk procedures for needlestick injuries; by using safer devices these can be reduced up to 76% (CDC 1997). In Europe, ten years later, the EU Council Directive 89/391/

EEC (1989) was amended with a new resolution for Safety and Health of Workers (EU 2006) which obligates employers to replace dangerous practices with the non-dangerous or the less dangerous. In 2010 a new EU Directive was issued (EU 2010). The directive sets out in EU law requirements for risk assessment, prevention and treatment of sharps injuries among healthcare workers. This legislation specifically addresses one of the priority objectives of the EU's current strategy for health and safety at work, which aims to cut workplace accidents by 25% by 2012 (EU 2010). The emphasis here is on both employers' and employees' responsibilities. Risk assessments are pivotal to achieving the aims of this legislation.

This EU legislation represents an important step toward acknowledging and supporting workers with the reality of their high-risk working practice, especially around sharps devices and body fluids. However, the EU legislation, unlike the USA Needlestick Safety and Prevention Act 2000 (USA 2000), does not yet make it mandatory for employers to evaluate, select and use engineering controls (e.g. sharps with engineered sharps injury protection or needle-free systems) to eliminate or minimise exposure to contaminated sharps.

CONCLUSION

This chapter has focused on equipment design in relation to practical use while offering detailed description to aid understanding behind design and intended use. Cannula development has been placed within a historical context to emphasise that while design and use of equipment has advanced significantly, there is still room for improvement. It is therefore hoped that the leaner will first learn how best to use equipment and then go on to question why it is designed and used in its current way. Future evolution will emerge from practitioners who can see ways to improve safety and quality to benefit patient, staff and the organisation.

REFERENCES AND FURTHER READING

CDC (1997) *Morbidity and Mortality Weekly Report*, 17 January.
CLSI – Clinical and Laboratory Standards Institute (USA) (2003) *Tubes and Additives for Venous Blood Specimen Collection; Approved Standards*, 5th edn. CLSI Document H1-A5.

CLSI Clinical and Laboratory Standards Institute (USA) (2004) *Procedures and Devices for the Collection of Diagnostic Capillary Blood Specimens: Approved Standards*, 5th edn. CLSI Document H4-A5.

CLSI – Clinical and Laboratory Standards Institute (USA) (2008) *Collection, Transport, and Processing of Blood Specimens for Testing Plasma-Based Coagulation Assays and Molecular Haemostasis Assays: Approved Guideline*, 5th edn. CLSI Document H21-A5.

CLSI: (2007) Procedures for the Collection of Diagnostic Blood Specimens by Venipuncture; Approved Standard – Sixth Edition; H3-A6; Volume 27, Number 26; CLSI: Wayne, Pennsylvania.

CLSI (2008): Clinical and Laboratory Standards Institute (USA): Collection, Transport, and processing of Blood Specimens for Testing Plasma-Based Coagulation Assays and molecular Haemostatis Assays; Approved Guideline-5th.

Corrigan, A. (2001) History of intravenous therapy. In: *Infusion Therapy in Clinical Practice* (eds J. Hankins, R.A. Waldman Lonsway, C. Hedrick & M. Perdue), 2nd edn. WB Saunders, Philadelphia.

Eucomed (2008) www.eucomed.be (accessed 8 August 2008).

EPINet Report 2001 (2003) *Advances in Exposure Prevention*, Vol. 6, No. 3.

EU (2006) Healthcare workers and blood-borne infections due to needlestick injuries. PE 374.502. European Parliament resolution with recommendations to the Commission on protecting European healthcare workers from blood-borne infections due to needlestick injuries (2006/2015(INI)) P6_TA(2006)0305.

EU (2010) Implementing the Framework Agreement on prevention from sharp injuries in the hospital and healthcare sector concluded by HOSPEEM and EPSU Council Directive 2010/32/EU. L134/68 May 2010.

Fitzgerald, M. & McIntosh, N. (1989) Pain and analgesia in the newborn. *Archives of Diseases in Childhood*, **64**, 441–443.

Garza, D. & Becan-McBride, K. (2002) *Blood Collection Equipment in Phlebotomy Handbook*. Pearson Education Inc, Upper Saddle River, NJ.

Gaukroger, P.B., Roberts, J.G. & Manners, T.A. (1988) Infusion thrombophlebitis: a prospective comparison of 645 Vialon and Teflon cannulae in anaesthetic and postoperative use. *Anaesthesia and Intensive Care*, **16**, 265–271.

HPA (2006) *Eye of the needle: United Kingdom surveillance of significant exposure to bloodborne viruses in healthcare workers*. Health Protection Agency.

Iserson, K.V. (1987) The origins of the gauge system for medical equipment. *Journal of Emergency Medicine*, **5**, 45–48.

International Organization for Standardization (1991) *ISO 9626: Stainless steel needle tubing for the manufacture of medical devices*. ISO, Geneva.

International Organization for Standardization (2001) *Amendment 1 to ISO 9626*. ISO, Geneva.

Jacquot, C., Fauvage, B., Bru, J.P., Croize, J. & Calop, J. (1989): Effect of type of material on thrombophlebitis risk with peripheral venous catheters. *Annales Françaises d'Anesthésie et de Réanimation*, **8**, 3–7.

Mainardi, G. (1743) *Bullarium Romanum*, III, iii (Rome, 1743), pp. 190–225.

Maki, D.G. & Ringer, M. (1991) Risk factors for infusion-related phlebitis with small peripheral venous catheters. *Annals of Internal Medicine*, **114**, 845–854.

Massa, D. (1951) A plastic needle. *Anaesthesiology*, **12**, 772–773.

McCall, R.E. & Tankersley, C.M. (2008) *Phlebotomy Essentials*, 4th edn. Lippincott Williams & Wilkins, Philadelphia.

McKee, J.M., Shell, J.A., Warren, T.A. & Campbell, V.P. (1989) Complications of intravenous therapy: a randomised prospective study – Vialon vs Teflon. *Journal of Intravenous Nursing*, **129**, 288–295.

MHRA (2001) *One Liners Issue* (November). No. 15.

NCCLS – National Committee for Clinical Laboratory Standards (1991) *Document H3-A3 Vol. II, No 10. Procedures for the Collection of Diagnostic Blood Specimens by Venepuncture*, 3rd edn. Section 6.19.

NCCLS – National Committee for Clinical Laboratory Standards (USA) (2006) *Procedures for the Collection of Diagnostic Blood Specimens by Skin Puncture. NCCLS Guidelines*, H3-A3, Vol. 11, No. 10.

Oberhammer, E.P. (1980) Contamination of injection ports on intravenous cannulae. *Lancet*, **ii**, 1027-1028.

Pilsworth, R. (1981) Risk from cannulae used to maintain intravenous access. *BMJ*, **282**, 222–223.

Rivera, A.M., Staruss, K.W., Zundert van, A. & Mortier, E. (2005) The history of peripheral intravenous catheters: How little plastic tubes revolutionized medicine. *Acta Anaesthesiologica Belgica*, **56**, 271–282.

Rivera, A.M., Strauss, K.W., Van Zundert, A.A.J. & Mortier, E.P. (2007) Matching the peripheral intravenous catheter to the individual patient. *Acta Anaesthesiologica Belgica*, **58**, 19–25.

Sommer, S.R., Warekois, R.S. & Robinson, R. (2002) *Venepuncture Equipment in Phlebotomy Workbook and Procedures Manual*. Saunders, Philadelphia.

Stanley, M.D., Meister, E. & Fuschuber, K. (1992) Infiltration during intravenous therapy in neonates: comparison of Teflon & Vialon catheters. *Southern Medical Journal*, **85**, 883–886.

Stankovic, A. & Smith, S. (2004) Elevated serum potassium values. *American Journal of Clinical Pathology*, **121**(Suppl. 1), S105–S112.

UNISON (1999) *Health and Safety Organiser*, Issue 6, December.

USA (2000) Needlestick Safety and Prevention Act.

Vein Selection

5

Barbara Witt

LEARNING OUTCOMES
The practitioner will be able to:
- ❏ Describe a suitable vein for venepuncture and cannulation.
- ❏ List five ways of encouraging a vein to dilate.
- ❏ Identify the type of veins to avoid for venepuncture and cannulation.
- ❏ Identify and discuss how mastectomy, axillary node dissection and radiotherapy to the axilla will affect venepuncture and cannulation.
- ❏ Know where to perform venepuncture if an intravenous (IV) infusion is in progress.
- ❏ Understand how age would impact on venepuncture and cannulation

INTRODUCTION
The practitioner plays a vital role in ensuring that procedures such as venepuncture and cannulation are performed safely, efficiently and as pain free as possible. Careful patient assessment and vein selection will help to achieve this. The practitioner can utilise various methods to improve venous access.

METHODS OF VEIN SELECTION
There are two key aspects to selecting a suitable vein:

1. visual inspection
2. palpation.

Venepuncture and Cannulation, first edition. Edited by Sarah Phillips,
Mary Collins and Lisa Dougherty. Published 2011 by Blackwell Publishing Ltd.
© 2011 Blackwell Publishing Ltd.

Visual inspection

Prior to applying the tourniquet to either arm the practitioner should visually assess the suitability of the arm. Visual inspection will enable the practitioner to avoid any areas of infection, phlebitis, oedema, bruised areas and sites that have been frequently used for venepuncture or cannulation.

Infection

Intact skin acts a barrier against infection but with the insertion of any intravenous device, which breaches the continuity of the skin, the patient is at an increased risk of infection (Hart 2008). The practitioner should therefore avoid any areas of infection or inflammation when selecting a site for venepuncture and cannulation.

Haematoma

A haematoma or bruise develops when blood leaks from a vein into the surrounding tissue during or after venepuncture and/ or cannulation (Ernst 2005). The practitioner should avoid areas of previous haematoma/bruising as this may be painful to the patient (McCall & Tankersley 2008). Also blood samples taken from this area may be contaminated with haemolysed blood that has leaked outside the vein (McCall & Tankersley 2008). Occasionally, if no other vein is suitable then venepuncture should be performed in an area that is distal to the haematoma (Hoeltke 2006).

Oedema

Access may be limited if the patient's arm is oedematous. A swollen arm can make palpation difficult. The application of a tourniquet may cause tissue damage and make indentations in the skin. The sample taken may also be contaminated with fluid (Hoeltke 2006).

Damaged skin

Areas of skin that have been burned or scarred should be avoided as palpation to these areas may be difficult. Burn sites that have healed may have impaired circulation, giving inaccurate blood results. Recently burned sites would be painful and predispose the patient to an increased risk of infection (McCall & Tankersley 2008). Scarring may be caused by numerous venepunctures, e.g. blood/apheresis donors. The veins may become hard, lose elasticity and make needle penetration more difficult (Ernst 2005). The practitioner should avoid areas with tattoos as circulation to these areas may be impaired and there may be an increased risk of infection. The dyes used in tattoos may also affect blood results (McCall & Tankersley 2008).

Palpation

Correct identification of a suitable vein for venepuncture or cannulation can only be determined by careful palpation. Palpation will enable the practitioner to identify the location, size, depth and condition of the vein and to avoid valves, arteries and tendons. It will also ensure that the correct type and size of device is selected. Palpation may prevent inadvertent insertion of the needle into other anatomical structures such as arteries, valves and tendons.

The practitioner should use the tip of the index finger on their less dominant hand to palpate the vein as this allows for re-palpation while realignment is performed using the dominant hand if the vein is missed. The practitioner should run their fingers smoothly over the selected site, gently pressing down and feeling for the rounded structure of the vein wall. The vein should feel soft and bouncy to the touch (Hoeltke 2006) and when depressed it should refill easily (Dougherty 2008). The practitioner should trace the path of the vein, palpating to determine the size, angle and depth of the vessel. If the vein is visible it may appear easier to access, especially for a new practitioner, but palpation is a more accurate method of ensuring the most suitable vessel has been selected. Skill in palpating a vein will improve with practice (Ernst 2005). Repeated use of the same fingers in palpation will improve sensitivity and the ability to distinguish veins and other structures (Weinstein 2007; Dougherty 2008). The thumb should not be used to palpate as it is less sensitive and has a pulse (Weinstein 2007). It may be useful to practise palpation on colleagues' veins as it will increase confidence in this method and reduce the reliance on sight.

Valves

Valves can be palpated in veins. Valves are formed by folds of endothelium and are usually observed or palpated as 'bulges' in the vein (Weinstein 2007). Valves tend to occur at points of branching or bifurcation, their function being to prevent the backflow of blood (Weinstein 2007). When performing venepuncture, the practitioner should insert the needle above the valve to prevent it from compressing and closing the lumen of the vein as this can make blood withdrawal difficult (Weinstein 2007; Dougherty 2008). For cannulation, the valve can make advancing the needle difficult and if forced can cause pain and damage to the vessel (Dougherty 2008).

Arteries

Arteries transport blood away from the heart and tend to be positioned more deeply than veins (Weinstein 2007). They also have much thicker walls and do not collapse if blood pressure falls (Weinstein 2007). Occasionally, patients may have an aberrant artery which is more superficial and sited in an unusual location (Weinstein 2007). An aberrant artery should not be mistaken for a vein. On palpation the practitioner should check the vessel for a pulse in order to identify if it is an artery. Arteries pulsate, veins do not. If an artery is punctured the patient may complain of severe pain and the practitioner may observe bright red blood (see Chapter 8). If a cannula is inadvertently placed in an artery and drugs are administered the patient may complain of severe pain during the infusion. It may cause arterial spasm and ischaemia leading to necrosis and gangrene of the limb (Weinstein 2007; Dougherty 2008).

Tendons

Tendons are bands of inelastic collagenous fibres and may have the appearance of a vein but on palpation they would feel hard to the touch (Hoeltke 2006).

Nerves

Nerve are neither visible nor palpable (Ernst 2005); they tend to lie deep in the tissues but sometimes they are close to the surface and will lie alongside veins and arteries. If a nerve is touched with a needle the patient will complain of a shooting 'electric shock' type pain and if the nerve is damaged, the nerve injury is often disabling and can be permanent (Ernst 2005) (see Chapter 8).

IMPROVING VENOUS ACCESS

There are numerous methods of improving venous access that the practitioner may consider:

- application of a tourniquet
- application of heat
- position of the limb
- fist clench/massage
- application of glyceryl trinitrate patches.

Application of a tourniquet

A tourniquet is used to increase the distension of veins when a sample of blood is being taken or when a cannula is being inserted. There are several types of tourniquet available. The choice may depend on personal preference and availability. A good quality, buckle closure, single hand release is most effective (Dimech *et al.* 2011). Consideration should be given to the type of material and the ability to decontaminate. There is a potential risk of cross-infection during peripheral venous access by contamination of tourniquets and the use of disposable tourniquets is recommended (Golder 2000). Consideration should be given to the use of latex-free tourniquets (RCN 2010).

A blood pressure cuff can be applied instead of a tourniquet (Ernst 2005). It may be more comfortable for the patient as the pressure is exerted over a wider area. The cuff should be inflated to a level just below the patient's diastolic level, or inflation to 40 mmHg is usually adequate (Hoeltke 2006). The practitioner should be able to reduce the pressure of the cuff easily following insertion of the needle.

The tourniquet should be applied around the upper forearm approximately 7–8 cm above the venepuncture site. It should be tight enough to impede venous return but not restrict arterial flow (McCall & Tankersley 2008). The tourniquet may be applied over a sleeve or a paper towel if there is a risk of causing injury or bruising to the skin, especially in elderly patients where the skin may be fragile (McCall & Tankersley 2008). Care should also be taken with thrombocytopenic patients or those on anti-coagulants (Dougherty 2008).

The tourniquet should not pinch the skin when tightened or be left on for more than one minute as the obstruction to blood flow may cause haemoconcentration and pooling of the blood leading to inaccurate blood results (Hoeltke 2006). A tightened tourniquet may also become uncomfortable for the patient if left on for an extended period of time.

It is suggested that after initial vein selection the tourniquet is not reapplied for at least two minutes to allow blood composition to return to normal (McCall & Tankersley 2008). The practitioner can utilise this time to prepare equipment and clean the skin.

Application of heat
The aim of applying heat is to increase vasodilation and improve venous filling. This method can be very effective in improving venous access. The practitioner can warm the venepuncture site by application of a heat pack or submerging the limb in warm water for a period of time. Research suggests that local warming facilitates the insertion of peripheral venous cannula, reducing both the time and number of attempts required (Lenhardt *et al.* 2002).

Position of the limb
Venous access can be improved by lowering the extremity below the level of the heart. The downward position allows gravity to help the vein to fill and become more prominent (Weinstein 2007). The arm should then be positioned comfortably on a pillow and straightened to help 'fix' the vein and make it easier to locate (McCall & Tankersley 2008).

Fist clench/massage

The patient may be asked to clench or make a fist, encouraging muscles to force blood into the veins and promote venous distension. Many patients prefer to clench on a washable hand grip, especially if they have long finger nails. The patient should be discouraged from vigorously squeezing the hand grip as this action may affect certain blood results, e.g. (Garza & Becan-McBride 2010). Light tapping of a vein may be useful but can be painful to the patient and cause the formation of haematoma in patients who have fragile veins, e.g. patients with thrombocytopenia (Dougherty 2008).

Application of glyceryl trinitrate patches

Small amounts of glyceryl trinitrate in patch form may be applied to improve local vasodilation and aid venepuncture (Weinstein 2007). Research suggests the application of glyceryl trinitrate will make cannulation easier (Hecker *et al.* 1983).

VEIN SELECTION

Basic anatomy will vary with each individual, so the numerous variations in vein position should be taken into consideration when selecting a vein (McCall & Tankersley 2008). See Tables 5.1 and 5.2.

'The triangular area in front of and slightly distal to the elbow is the cubital or antecubital fossa' (Monkhouse 2007). This is

Table 5.1 Suitability of veins for venepuncture and cannulation

Suitable veins should be:	Veins to avoid are:
Soft	Hard
Bouncy	Thrombosed
Well supported	Thin
Easily palpable	Fragile
Straight	Mobile
	Overlying bony prominence, e.g. inner aspect of the wrist

Table 5.2 Location of veins

Digital veins	May be used for venepuncture	May be cannulated as a last resort for fluid replacement
Metacarpal veins	Acceptable for venepuncture	Suitable for cannulation/short term IV therapy
Medial veins/ antecubital fossa	Ideal for venepuncture	Not suitable for routine cannulation
Cephalic vein		Ideal for cannulation
Basilic vein		Often overlooked; valves make advancement of cannula difficult
Dorsal venous network of the foot	May be used for venepuncture but increased risk of complications	Increased risk of complications Doctor's consent may be required

where the most suitable veins for venepuncture are located. The veins are superficial, usually visible and easily palpable. The basilic, median cubital and cephalic veins, pass through this area. The cephalic vein rises from the dorsal veins and flows upwards on the lateral (outside) aspect of the arm. The basilic vein has its origins in the ulnar border of the hand and forearm and lies on the medial (inner) aspect of the arm (Waugh & Grant 2010) (see Chapter 2).

The median cubital vein is the most suitable for venepuncture because it is:

- superficial and easy to palpate
- well supported
- offers less risk of injury to underlying structures (Ernst 2005).

However, the antecubital fossa is not suitable for cannulation because of joint flexion which may increase the risk of mechanical irritation resulting in phlebitis (Weinstein 2007) and can increase the risk of the cannula being dislodged (Dougherty 2008).

Cephalic vein

The cephalic vein provides an excellent vein for cannulation owing to its size and location. Care must be taken to avoid the radial nerve (Scales 2008).

Basilic vein

The basilic vein can appear prominent but is not well supported and tends to 'roll', which makes venepuncture and cannulation difficult (McCall & Tankersley 2008). Also, because of its location there is an increased risk of haematoma formation if the patient flexes the arm when the needle is removed (Weinstein 2007). Numerous valves may be present, which can make advancement of a cannula difficult (Dougherty 2008). Care must be taken to avoid accidental puncture of the median cutaneous nerve and brachial artery, which are in close proximity (McCall & Tankersley 2008).

Veins of the hand

The metacarpal veins are often used for venepuncture when veins in the antecubital fossa are not accessible. The metacarpal veins may appear prominent but are not always well supported and tend to 'roll', especially in elderly patients (Hoeltke 2006). If using a metacarpal vein the practitioner should choose a smaller gauge needle, e.g. 23G, and ensure that the vein is anchored securely on insertion. The metacarpal veins are often a good option for cannulation and short-term intravenous therapy. The bones of the hand provide a natural splint and help to secure the device (Scales 2008).

Veins of the feet

Occasionally, if no alternative sites are available, it may be necessary to perform a venepuncture or cannulation on the lower extremities. However, veins in the lower extremities should not routinely be used in adults due to the risk of complications (RCN 2010). Venepuncture or cannulation is contraindicated in the feet if the patient is diabetic or has a previous history of deep vein thrombosis or coagulation disorders (for paediatrics see later section).

Prior to performing venepuncture or cannulation on a lower extremity the practitioner should ensure the organisation has a policy to support this procedure or if approval/consent is required by the doctor and the patient (Ernst 2005; Hoeltke 2006). Cannulation in the lower extremities is usually avoided due to the risk of complications such as thrombophlebitis and pulmonary embolus (Weinstein 2007). The blood flow within an extremity should be considered when selecting a site for cannulation. The infusion of non-irritant drugs into a vein with low blood flow may be acceptable (Scales 2008) but this may lead to pooling of infused drugs and raised concentration levels or delay to the required effect of a medication (Weinstein 2007). If the cannula is required for the administration of irritant solutions and there is no other available access then consideration should be given to the use of a central venous access device (Scales 2008). A cannula sited in a lower extremity should always be re-sited as soon as a more suitable vein is available. (Dougherty 2008).

The veins used for access in the lower extremities are those found on the dorsum of the foot and the saphenous vein of the ankle. Veins in the ankle tend to 'roll' and the practitioner may find access easier if the patient extends the foot to secure the vein (Garza & Becan-McBride 2005).

The veins of the feet and ankles are often smaller in diameter so the practitioner must select a small gauge device (Ernst 2005). Consideration should be given to the individual's ability to mobilise if a cannula is sited in the foot.

FACTORS THAT MAY AFFECT CHOICE FOR VENEPUNCTURE AND CANNULATION

Cerebrovascular accident (CVA)
The placement of a needle into the affected limb of a patient who has suffered a CVA is contraindicated. The patient may have reduced or absent neurological sensation in the limb which could prevent the patient from detecting any pain (Dougherty 2008). Reduced mobility and restricted movement may also make it difficult for the patient to hyperextend their arm and make access to the antecubital fossa difficult (Ernst

2005). The practitioner should perform venepuncture and cannulation on the unaffected limb. Careful vein selection is required with consideration to the possibility of rotating the choice of site selected to prevent repeated use and scarring. The practitioner needs to ensure that all equipment is placed within reach as the patient would be unable to assist, i.e. when asked to apply pressure when the needle is removed.

Parkinson's disease

It may be difficult to perform venepuncture or cannulation on a patient with Parkinson's disease because of the movement and tremors of the fingers and limbs (McCall & Tankersley 2008). The practitioner should ensure the limb is well supported and may need to request help in holding or supporting the limb. The practitioner should be aware of the risk of needlestick injury that could be caused by the uncontrolled movement.

Surgery or radiotherapy to the axilla

Prior to commencing venepuncture or cannulation the practitioner should ascertain whether the patient has received surgery or radiotherapy to the axilla. Patients with breast cancer who have received treatment are the most obvious to consider but the practitioner also needs to review melanoma and lymphoma patients. Axillary node dissection may cause lymphostasis, predisposing the patient to an increased risk of infection (Garza & Becan-McBride 2010). No tourniquet or blood pressure cuff should be applied to the ipsilateral (affected) arm as this may lead to injury. Venepuncture and/ or cannulation should be performed on the contralateral (unaffected) arm (Cole 2006). If the patient has had bilateral treatment the practitioner should refer to local hospital policy regarding use of the ipsilateral arm. Some hospitals will require consent from the doctor while others will require the patient to sign a consent form once they have received information on the risk factors. The RCN *Standards for Infusion Therapy* (2010) states that 'the patient, caregiver or legally authorised representative should be informed of potential complications associated with treatment or therapy'.

If the patient has had bilateral surgery/axillary radiotherapy the practitioner should consider:

- selecting a vein in the lower extremities (depending on hospital policy)
- selecting the limb that was treated first
- selecting the limb that received surgery but no radiotherapy
- selecting the patient's non-dominant arm.

The practitioner may also need to consider the type of treatment, i.e. curative versus palliative. If access is to be long term then consideration should be given to the insertion of a central venous access device and this should be discussed with the patient.

Arteriovenous fistula
A patient who has undergone dialysis may have an arteriovenous fistula sited. An arteriovenous fistula is an artificial shunt which permanently fuses a vein and artery. The connection is usually close to the surface of the skin and the formed loop is easy to visualise and feel. The practitioner should never apply a tourniquet or blood pressure cuff to this area and venepuncture and/or cannulation should be avoided as this could predispose the patient to problems if the site becomes infected (Ernst 2005). The practitioner should use an alternative site.

Intravenous (IV) infusion in progress
If a patient has an intravenous infusion in progress, the practitioner should avoid using this arm for venepuncture. Any blood samples taken above an IV infusion may be contaminated with the IV solution and either cause the blood samples to be diluted or cause an elevation in the results depending on the type of additive, e.g. potassium (Ernst 2005) This can have serious ramifications for the patient; the Serious Hazard of Transfusion (SHOT) *Annual Report 2006* (SHOT 2007) reports on an 80-year-old woman who died from cardiac failure following an unnecessary transfusion which was based on a haemoglobin of 3.9 g/dL. Investigation showed that the blood sample with a haemoglobin of 3.9 g/dL was diluted by an intravenous infusion.

If the practitioner cannot take blood from the opposite arm, she/he should consider the following:

1. *Blood sample collection below the infusion site, e.g. metacarpal vein.* As the infusion is flowing upwards any blood taken below the infusion should not be contaminated. There is therefore no requirement to discard any blood or switch off the infusion, although some authors suggest that the infusion should be switched off and the first 5 mL of blood be discarded (Ernst 2005; Hoeltke 2006). However, if this option is followed it should be documented on the blood request form.

2. *Blood sample collection above the infusion site.* Occasionally, the practitioner may need to consider performing venepuncture above the IV infusion. The practitioner should refer to local policy regarding this option and follow the procedure for turning off an infusion and maintaining patency during the procedure. Consideration should be given to the type of infusion in progress as local policy may exclude the disruption of some types of infusion depending on the additives (Ernst 2005). If this option is to be followed, the practitioner must consult with nursing staff caring for the patient regarding discontinuing the infusion. Then if it is appropriate, the device should be flushed to ensure patency and left for 10–15 minutes. The blood can then be taken as per normal routine (ideally in an alternative vein to the infusion). It should be documented on the request form that the sample was taken above an IV infusion that had been temporarily discontinued. The infusion should then be recommenced.

Children

Venepuncture and cannulation in neonates and children should only be performed by skilled and experienced practitioners (Ernst 2005). The procedure will require time, patience and an understanding of child development. Children's veins tend to be smaller and hidden by subcutaneous fat (Bravery 2008). Children may be less cooperative and have fears about the equipment, e.g. needles linked to previous experiences and observation (Ernst 2005; Hoeltke 2006). The practitioner plays an important role in allaying the child's fears and gaining trust and cooperation. The practitioner should always be honest, speak at eye level and use words that are appropriate for that particular age group (Garza & Beacon-McBride 2010).

Role play and the use of toys may assist in the explanation of equipment and procedures. Providing bravery certificates and badges may also encourage cooperation (Hoeltke 2006). Parents should be encouraged to comfort and support the child. Specialised equipment should be used where available, i.e. winged infusion device for venepuncture.

Choice of veins

Scalp veins (infants or toddler)
Scalp veins may be selected when alternative veins are difficult or unsuitable. Scalp veins tend to be superficial and easily visualised until approximately 12–18 months when the hair follicles mature and the superficial layers of skin thicken (Weinstein 2007). A flat rubber band may be applied around the head as a tourniquet (Garza & Becan-McBride 2010). The practitioner should ensure that the infant is kept warm throughout the procedure. Occasionally it may be necessary to shave the scalp, which may cause additional distress to the family and consent must be obtained prior to this being undertaken (Weinstein 2007). A benefit of using the scalp vein is that it enables the child to have free hands for movement and to allow thumb sucking (Bravery 2008).

Feet (infant/toddler)
The veins in the foot can be large and accessible but it may prove difficult to maintain a cannulation device on an active mobile toddler (Bravery 2008).

Hand and arm veins (toddler – adolescent)
These are the most commonly used sites for peripheral venous access in children (Bravery 2008). On infants the dorsal hand veins can be accessed without the application of a tourniquet. The practitioner should use their middle finger and forefinger to encircle the wrist and apply pressure (Hoeltke 2006). Veins in the antecubital fossa can be difficult to access in babies or toddlers due to subcutaneous fat.

Improving venous access

The practitioner can improve venous dilation by encouraging the child to play in warm water. The use of a venoscope transluminator (which emits a high density light that illuminates the vein) may be beneficial (Hoeltke 2006). Consideration should always be given to the choice of limb, movement and the ability to allow thumb sucking (Weinstein 2007).

Older people

When performing venepuncture or cannulation on older patients the practitioner needs to take certain factors into consideration.

Skin

The natural ageing process will bring changes to the depth, texture and integrity of the skin (Fabian 2009).The epidermis (outer layer) becomes thinner with decreased healing and barrier protection. The dermis (middle layer), which incorporates the blood vessels and nerves, decreases in thickness with a reduction in the number of nerve endings and sweat glands. The practitioner should be aware of the patient's decreased level of sensation when performing venepuncture and cannulation (Fabian 2009) Diminished skin turgor and the decrease in the amount of subcutaneous tissue can make venepuncture and cannulation difficult as the veins are less supported and have a tendency to 'roll'. These veins will need to be anchored securely (Dougherty 2008). As the skin may be thin and fragile the practitioner should also be cautious with the type of tape used to secure any device and alternative methods may need to be implemented (Fabian 2009). Blood vessels will lose elasticity and become more fragile with an increased risk of haematoma formation occurring during and after the procedure (Ernst 2005; McCall & Tankersley 2008).

Musculoskeletal

The onset of arthritis can leave joints swollen and painful, which can make venous access difficult. The patient may have restricted movement and have difficulty in extending an arm or opening a hand (McCall & Tankersley 2008). The practitioner should avoid using areas of flexion as this could cause restricted movement to an arthritic joint (Fabian 2009). The patient should be involved in ensuring a comfortable position is established prior to selecting a venepuncture and cannulation site (McCall & Tankersley 2008).

Sensory (visual and hearing)

The practitioner should ensure that the patient is fully aware of the procedure when performing venepuncture and cannulation. Hearing impaired patients may require the practitioner to speak slowly and clearly, using a pen and paper if necessary. For visual loss the practitioner should avoid using hand gestures and explain verbally the procedure as it is performed (McCall & Tankersley 2008).

Mental impairment

Older people may suffer from conditions such as dementia or Alzheimer disease. The practitioner may need to liaise with a relative or caregiver for information. The practitioner should appreciate that the patient may feel anxious or confused and should approach the patient in a calm, confident manner and use simple explanations (McCall & Tankersley 2008).

CONCLUSION

The key to successful venepuncture or cannulation is good vein selection. By selecting the right vein, in a suitable condition and appropriate location, the practitioner will have more chance of first time success; careful selection of a vein will lead to a less painful experience for the patient and ensure better cannula dwell time.

REFERENCES

Bravery, K. (2008) Paediatric intravenous therapy in practice. In: *Intravenous Therapy in Nursing Practice* (eds L. Dougherty & J. Lamb), 2nd edn. Blackwell Publishing, Oxford.

Cole, T. (2006) Risks and benefits of needle use in patients after axillary node surgery. *British Journal of Nursing*, **15**(18), 969–979.

Dimech, A et al. (2011) Venepuncture. In: *The Royal Marsden Manual of Clinical Procedures* (eds L. Dougherty & S. Lister), 8th edn, Blackwell Publishing, Oxford.

Dougherty, L. (2008) Obtaining peripheral access. In: *Intravenous Therapy in Nursing Practice* (eds L. Dougherty & J. Lamb), 2nd edn. Blackwell Publishing, Oxford.

Ernst, D. (2005) *Applied Phlebotomy*. Lippincott Williams & Wilkins, Philadelphia.

Fabian, B. (2009) Infusion therapy in the older adult. In: *Infusion Nursing: An Evidence Based Approach* (eds M. Alexander *et al.*), 3rd edn, pp. 571–582. WB Saunders, Philadelphia.

Finlay, T. (2004) Vascular access devices. In: *Intravenous Therapy. Essential Clinical Skills for Nurses*. Blackwell Publishing, Oxford.

Garza, D. & Becan-McBride, K. (2002) *Phlebotomy Handbook. Blood Collection Essentials*. Prentice Hall, Upper Saddle River, NJ.

Garza, D. & Becan-McBride, K. (2005) *Phlebotomy Handbook. Blood Collection Essentials*, 7th edn. Pearson Prentice Hall, Upper Saddle River, NJ.

Garza, D. & Becan-McBride, K. (2010) *Phlebotomy Handbook. Blood Collection Essentials*, 8th edn. Pearson, Upper Saddle River, NJ.

Golder, M. (2000) Potential risk of cross infection during peripheral venous access by contamination of tourniquets. *Lancet*, **355**, 44.

Hart, S., (2008) Infection Control. *Intravenous Therapy in Nursing Practice*. (eds L. Dougherty & J. Lamb), 2nd edn, 89. Blackwell Publishing, Oxford.

Hecker, J.F., Lewis B.H. & Stanley, H. (1983) Nitroglycerine ointment as an aid to venepuncture. *Lancet* **1**, 202–206.

Hoeltke, L.B. (2006) *The Complete Textbook of Phlebotomy*, 3rd edn. Thomson Delmar Learning, New York.

Lenhardt, R., Seybold, T., Kimberger, O., Stoiser, B. & Sessler, D.I. (2002) Local warming and insertion of peripheral venous cannulas: single blinded prospective randomised controlled trial and single blinded randomised crossover trial. *British Medical Journal*, **325**, 409–412.

McCall, R.E. & Tankersley, C.M. (2008) *Phlebotomy Essentials*. Lippincott Williams & Wilkins, Philadelphia.

Monkhouse, S. (2007) Upper limb. In: *Master Medicine: Clinical Anatomy*, 2nd edn. Churchill Livingstone Elsevier, Edinburgh.

RCN (2010) *Standards for Infusion Therapy*. Royal College of Nursing, London.

Scales, K. (2008) Anatomy and physiology related to intravenous therapy. In: *Intravenous Therapy in Nursing Practice* (eds L. Dougherty & J. Lamb), 2nd edn, pp. 23–48. Blackwell Publishing, Oxford.

SHOT – Serious Hazards of Transfusion (2007) *Annual Report 2006*, p. 17. http://www.shotuk.org/SHOT_report_2006.pdf (accessed 11 January 2010).

Waugh, A. & Grant, A. (2010) The cardiovascular system. In: *Anatomy and Physiology in Health and Illness*, 11th edn, p. 101. Churchill Livingstone, Edinburgh.

Weinstein, S. (2007) *Plumer's Principles and Practice of Intravenous Therapy*, 8th edn. Lippincott Williams & Wilkins, Philadelphia.

Witt, B. (2008) Venepuncture. In: *The Royal Marsden Manual of Clinical Procedures* (eds L. Dougherty & S. Lister),7th edn, pp. 919–931. Blackwell Publishing, Oxford.

6 | Infection Control and Risk Management

Sarah Hart

LEARNING OUTCOMES

The practitioner will be able to:

❑ Have an understanding of factors that predispose the patient to infection.

❑ Identify specific factors to venepuncture and cannulation including cleaning of the site, dressings, routine replacement of cannulae and administration sets.

❑ Discuss the implications of *Saving Lives* and other relevant recommendations.

❑ List how to prevent needlestick injuries.

❑ Describe the management of specimen handling and transportation.

INTRODUCTION

Prevalence surveys of healthcare acquired infection (HAI) estimate that 9% of patients will acquire an infection during their illness (Taylor *et al.* 2001). During medical and nursing care intravenous devices are indispensable as intravenous therapy is one of the commonest invasive procedure undertaken in hospital (Gabriel 2006). Regrettably 60% of bloodstream infections are related to intravenous devices (Department of Health 2003a). Furthermore whilst invasive procedures predispose the patient to HAIs, they also carry a risk to the healthcare worker under-

Venepuncture and Cannulation, first edition. Edited by Sarah Phillips,
Mary Collins and Lisa Dougherty. Published 2011 by Blackwell Publishing Ltd.
© 2011 Blackwell Publishing Ltd.

taking the procedure, who may experience a needlestick injury or contamination to mucous membranes or non-intact skin. This chapter highlights the importance of infection control and prevention, for both the patient and the healthcare worker, when performing venepuncture and cannulation.

INFECTION CONTROL

Healthcare acquired infections (HAI) are a leading cause of morbidity and mortality among hospitalised patients (Eggimann *et al.* 2004). Bloodstream infections accounted for 12% of all HAIs reported in a European Nosocomial Infection Surveillance system in the intensive care setting. (Vincent *et al.* 1995). Most bloodstream infections were associated with intravenous devices. The incidence of infection varies depending on the type of device, frequency of manipulation and the patient's risk factors. Rates are highest with central venous catheters and less so among those with peripheral devices (Vincent *et al.* 1995). An Australian study indicated a bacteraemia rate of 1 per 3000 cannulae (Collignon 1994). A more recent review found an infection rate of 0.2 per 1000 intravenous cannula days (McLaws & Taylor 2003). As peripheral devices are the most frequently used intravenous device, it does mean there is a significant risk of infection, with serious infectious complications that produce considerable annual morbidity (CDC 2002).

No single factor accounts for why a patient acquires an infection; however, factors that have been found to predispose the patient to infection include:

1. the patient themselves
2. the environment
3. healthcare workers' technique, including:
   * aseptic technique
   * hand washing
   * preparation of the patient
   * education and training.

The patient
Some patients have an increased vulnerability to HAIs due to a number of factors:

- Serious diseases, such as cancer or leukaemia, and transplantation procedures, causing the patient to become immunocompromised.
- Treatments such as steroids, radiotherapy and cytotoxic chemotherapy, which often damage the immune system as well as treating the cancer. This means during treatment and for sometime afterwards the patient is significantly immunosuppressed.
- Age, in the young patient due to their developing immune systems and the older person owing to their waning immune system.
- Invasive procedures, in particular surgery, urinary catheterisation and intravenous devices.
- Length of stay in hospital; the longer the hospital stay, the greater the exposure to pathogenic hospital microorganisms.
- Use of antibiotics, which leads to an alteration in the patient's normal flora. Antibiotics may kill or suppress the drug-sensitive microorganisms, whilst at the same time allowing the naturally drug-resistant organisms to survive and multiply. Patients who have developed an HAI caused by antimicrobial-resistant microorganisms will have an infection that will be more difficult to treat, and may result in an illness that is increased in length and severity, resulting in a longer inpatient stay.
- Patients often develop an infection from their own normal bacterial flora; this is referred to as endogenous infection (Hart 2006).

The hospital environment

The hospital environment must be visibly clean, free from dust and soilage and acceptable to patients, their visitors and staff (Department of Health 2008). Cleaning and disinfection programmes and protocols for environmental surfaces in patient care areas must be defined and areas fully monitored to ensure high standards of cleanliness are achieved (Department of Health 2003a). Whilst cleaning is everyone's responsibility (Jeanes 2005), the 'Modern Matron' (Department of Health 2003b) must lead by example and make changes when cleaning standards are not satisfactory.

High standards of cleanliness will help to reduce the risk of infection (RCN 2005a). A prospective study evaluating MRSA contamination of the environment found that even after routine cleaning, contamination persists, highlighting the need for effective cleaning (Sexton *et al.* 2006).

Patient areas must be cleaned daily and more often if contamination occurs. Equipment, such as drip stands and commodes that are often not included in the general cleaning staff duties, must be cleaned following each and every patient use by the ward staff. Infection control must be a consideration during planning, building or refurbishment of clinical areas, so that the environment is easily cleaned (National Health Service Estates 2002).

Healthcare workers' technique

Aseptic technique

Aseptic means without microorganisms. Aseptic technique is the process of reducing the risk of infection by decreasing the likelihood that microorganisms will contaminate a susceptible person. This may be the patient during an invasive procedure, or the healthcare worker who may be exposed to potentially infectious blood and body fluids during invasive procedures. An aseptic technique must be used during venepuncture, cannulation and during any aspect of care and management of the cannula entry site and infusion system (Dougherty & Watson 2008).

As aseptic technique is used for different procedures, by healthcare workers in variety of environments, two alternative aseptic techniques have emerged (Preston 2005). Firstly, a surgical aseptic technique which is generally used in the operating theatre, but can also be used in the ward for invasive procedures such as insertion of central venous catheters. A surgical aseptic technique involves hand washing using a full surgical scrub technique, use of sterile gown gloves and drapes.

Secondly, a technique that is used more commonly in the ward area is the non-touch aseptic technique or clean technique (Hart 2007), which is achieved either by using gloves or forceps to handle equipment that has been processed and sterilised in a central sterile service department or by using sterile disposable equipment (Ayliffe *et al.* 2002).

Aseptic technique includes:

1. hand washing
2. using sterile equipment
3. preparing the patient for the procedure
4. maintaining a sterile field during the procedure
5. maintaining an infection-free safe environment during the procedure.

Hand washing

Hand washing before and after every patient contact has been seen to reduce the risk of cross-infection (Christiaens *et al.* 2006). Sleeves should be rolled up, jewellery removed, nails should be kept short and clean, and nail varnish and false nails should not be worn in the clinical area. Cuts and abrasions must be covered with a waterproof dressing (Department of Health 2001).

A review by Kampf & Kramer (2004) of the solutions used for hand washing found that:

- plain soap and water has the lowest antimicrobial efficacy.
- alcohol-based handrubs have a broad and immediate antimicrobial efficacy against viruses and bacteria.
- alcohol-based handrubs are not effective in removing dirt or soiling.
- chlorhexidine and triclosan detergents are slower and less effective than alcohol.
- alcohol-based handrubs are also less irritating than soap and detergent and therefore have increased user acceptability.

Another study comparing alcohol-based handrubs with other products found that alcohol-based handrubs were more effective in removing microorganisms (Sickbert-Bennett *et al.* 2005). Furthermore, a quantitative study that assessed the introduction of alcohol-based handrubs found a 21% decrease in healthcare-acquired methicillin resistant *Staphylococcus aureus* (MRSA) and a 41% decrease in vancomycin-resistant enterococcus (VRE), but no change in *Clostridium difficile* levels (Gordin *et al.* 2005).

Hands should be washed with soap or detergent and warm water, rinsed and dried carefully with disposable paper towels when coming on duty. As long as hands do not become soiled, clean hands can then be decontaminated with alcohol-based handrub before and after every patient contact. Prior to beverage and meal breaks and when going home, hands should be washed with plain soap and water.

Using sterile equipment

Sterile equipment must be used during venepuncture and cannulation.

Sterilisation is a process used to render the object free from viable microorganisms, including bacterial spores and viruses. For reusable surgical equipment sterilisation will be undertaken in a central sterilisation department, using mechanical washing machines and steam autoclaves. Disposable equipment will be supplied sterile by the manufacturers; generally sterilisation is by irradiation. Single-use disposable items must never be cleaned and reused (National Health Service Estates 2003).

Preparing the patient

Informed consent

The patient must be fully informed of the procedure that is to be undertaken and give consent. This allows the patient to make an informed decision about their care (Scott *et al.* 2003), which will encourage the patient to cooperate with care (McParland *et al.* 2000). For example, uncooperative patients during cannulation and venepuncture may make sudden movements that could lead to a breach in the aseptic technique or to an inoculation accident.

Skin disinfection prior to invasive procedures

Correct skin preparation reduces the risk of infection by lowering the chances that bacteria from the patient's skin will contaminate the venepuncture or cannulation site.

Skin must be carefully cleaned prior to cannulation and venepuncture, as skin is colonised with a wide range of microorganisms, which have an impact on the incidence of intravenous device infections (Hadaway 2003). If the skin is visibly soiled it must be washed with detergent and warm water and carefully rinsed and dried. To clean the skin, solutions should be applied with friction using back and forth strokes for at least 30 seconds and alllowed to air dry for 30–60 seconds. The solution can be applied using non-linting sterile cotton wool, guaze swabs or using a sponge applicator, e.g. Frepp (Dougherty & Watson 2011). Once the skin is cleaned it must not be touched; if it is necessary to re-palpate, the skin must be re-cleaned (Dougherty & Watson 2008).

An antiseptic must be used to clean the skin; this will reduce the number of microorganisms without causing damage or irritation. In addition, some antiseptics can prevent the growth of microorganisms on the cleaned area for some time following cleaning. Chlorhexidine gluconate is effective against a broad range of microorganisms and has the added advantage of having a persistent effect by remaining effective for 4–6 hours (Pratt et al. 2007). A prospective study to assess the efficacy of cutaneous antisepsis to prevent catheter-associated infection found that 2% chlorhexidine substantially reduced the incidence of catheter-related infections (Maki et al. 1991). A more recent study of skin disinfectant prior to venepuncture found that 70% isopropyl alcohol was a convenient, low cost and tolerated skin cleansing agent (Calfee & Far 2002) as an alternative to chlorhexidine. However, the Department of Health (2007a, b) have recommended the use of 2% chlorhexidine to clean skin prior to cannulation and venepuncture when taking blood cultures.

Antiseptics are designed to reduce or destroy microorganisms on skin and must not be used to disinfect instruments. Care must be taken not to contaminate the disinfectant. The cotton wool or gauze must not be dipped into the main antiseptic container; instead a small amount of antiseptic should be poured into a sterile gallipot or poured directly onto the cotton wool or gauze, making sure not to touch the lip of the container on the cotton wool, gauze or gallipot. A used piece of cotton wool or gauze must not be put back with the unused items but should be disposed of into a clinical waste bag.

Skin preparation

Shaving of the skin prior to cannulation should be avoided as shaving can damage the epidermal layer which is a natural barrier against opportunistic microorganisms. A systematic review of 20 clinical studies that dealt with preoperative hair removal recommended that if hair removal is required, clipping or a depilatory cream should be used (Kjonniksen *et al.* 2002). These studies are supported by a more recent review which found the use of clippers superior to hair removal by razors (Niel-Weise *et al.* 2005).

Maintaining a sterile field

A sterile field is the area produced by the use of sterile towels to provide a working surface to hold the sterile equipment required during an aseptic technique.

Only sterile equipment is free from microorganisms. Once a sterile object comes into contact with a non-sterile object it is no longer sterile. Sterility can be maintained by the following means:

- Carefully open sterile packs so as not to contaminate them.
- Only place sterile items on the sterile field.
- Use sterile gloves or forceps to handle sterile items within the sterile field.
- Do not return used items to the sterile field.
- Do not open a sterile pack by an open window or door, or create excessive movement that may cause dust to settle on the sterile field.
- Carefully dispense supplementary items and liquids onto the sterile field or into sterile gallipots.
- When in doubt about the sterility of an item or area, consider it to be contaminated.
- Store equipment safely as MRSA can survive on sterile packs for many weeks (Dietze *et al.* 2001).

Other factors that reduce the risk of infection

Resiting of peripheral vascular devices

The longer a peripheral device is in place, the greater the risk of infection. There is very little difference between infection rates of devices left in for 72 hours compared with 96 hours. Therefore devices should be rotated at 72–96-hour intervals, but sooner if infection such as tenderness at the insertion site or fever without obvious cause is suspected (CDC 2002).

Replacement of administration sets

Replace administration sets every 72 hours unless catheter-related infection is suspected, or:

- every 24 hours when total parenteral nutrition is being administered
- every 12 hours or after every second unit of blood and on completion of the blood transfusion (British Committee for Standards in Haematology 1999).

Dressings

Following venepuncture a plaster is normally applied. When pressure needs to be applied a gauze swab and strapping is a suitable alternative.

A randomised study comparing gauze and transparent dressings for peripheral intravenous catheter sites found a trend towards lower frequencies of phlebitis and infiltration using the transparent dressing; this study also found that following cannulation transparent semi-permeable dressings were a suitable cannula dressing by reliably securing the device, allowing continuous inspection which requires infrequent changing (Tripepi-Bova et al. 1997), as well as allowing the patient to shower or bath without wetting the dressing (CDC 2002).

Education

All healthcare professionals who have clinical responsibility for patients should receive mandatory training as part of their induction and on an ongoing basis (RCN 2005a). Educational interventions for nurses and doctors have been shown to reduce the incidence of catheter-related bloodstream infections (Warren et al. 2003). Self-study modules for nurses related to handling intravenous devices have been found to be useful in helping to reduce infection rates (Eggimann et al. 2004). Competencies for capillary blood sampling and venepuncture in children and young children provide a framework so that practitioners can develop and maintain the ability to undertake these tasks (RCN 2005b).

Well-trained skilled healthcare workers are more likely to complete a task correctly and carefully. Unskilled workers are more likely to be clumsy, rough or undertake excessive manipulation which can damage the patient's tissues and cause bleeding, this damage to the tissue delays healing and predisposes the patient to infection. After a brief tutorial on the use of an ultrasound placement system it was found that nurses were able to successfully place peripheral intravenous devices in patients with difficult veins, thereby reducing the need for these patients to receive central venous access (Blaivas & Lyon 2006).

Saving Lives: Reducing Infection, Delivering Clean and Safe Care: High Impact Interventions (*Department of Health 2007a, b)*

These care bundles include good practice actions. There are two related to venepuncture and cannulation. One is concerned with insertion and ongoing care of peripheral cannulae (Department of Health 2007a) and the other with taking blood culture samples (Department of Health 2007b). They provide clear guidelines on appropriate elements of care that need to be achieved to prevent infection. The care bundles also include a tool to identify if all elements have or have not been achieved by organisations which enable improvement to be made.

Needlestick injuries

Needlestick injuries are a common occupational occurrence. The Health Protection Agency (2005b) has a reporting scheme that includes 150 centres. A cumulative total of 2140 reports were received between 1996 and 2004. Of these 47% involved hepatitis C reports, 26% HIV reports, 9% hepatitis B reports and 9% were accidents with patients who had dual and triple infections. In those cases where the report stated the location of the accident, 45% were in wards, 15% in the operating theatre, 11% accident and emergency departments, 8% in intensive care. The procedure during which most needlestick accidents occurred was recorded as being during venepuncture (17%).

Box 6.1 Prevention of needlestick injuries initiatives

1. Healthcare workers receive adequate training and education on the management and prevention of accidents.
2. All hospitals to have policies and procedures in place including what to do if an accident occurs.
3. Services in place to manage accidents quickly and efficiently.
4. Training, adoption and use of universal precautions.
5. Correct handling and disposal of used needles.
6. Provision of and training in use of personal protective equipment (PPE). In particular wearing and changing gloves between patients when undertaking invasive procedures.
7. Readily accessible and not overfilled puncture-resistant sharps containers.
8. Not resheathing used needles.
9. Washing hands before and after every patient contact.
10. Covering skin lesions with a waterproof plaster.
11. Management follow-up of all accidents to ensure that the appropriate action was taken (Department of Health 2004).
12. Introduction of needleless systems and intravenous safety devices (Marini *et al.* 2004).
13. Education, training and supervision.
14. Clinical governance follow-up of all accidents to establish whether changes in practices are required (Health Protection Agency 2005a).

Percutaneous injury is the most common reported accident in the UK, with nursing staff reporting most incidents (45%) followed by medical and dental staff (37%) (Health Protection Agency 2005b). There were nine incidents of hepatitis C seroconversion following a percutaneous exposure reported during 1996–2004 in the UK. Of these nine cases, six occurred following the procedure and five of these were preventable (see Box 6.1) (Health Protection Agency 2005b).

The first documented seroconversion after a specific exposure to HIV was reported in 1984. Since that time 106 cases have been reported worldwide, four of which were in the UK: one case in 1984 and three cases in 1992/3. There is also the possibility that a further 238 seroconversions may have been occupationally acquired (see Table 6.1), 14 of which were reported in the UK during 1984–1997. Included in these data are 24 cases of HIV seroconversion despite initiation of post-exposure prophylaxis (Health Protection Agency 2005a).

Table 6.1 Percentages of the disciplines of healthcare workers involved in documented and probable cases of occupationally acquired HIV

Healthcare worker	Percentage of documented cases	Percentage of probable cases
Nurses and clinical laboratory workers	69%	39%
Doctors	13%	12%
Surgeons	Less than 1%	7%
Dentists and dental workers	3%	

Source: Health Protection Agency (2005a).

Factors that increase the risk of acquiring HIV has been identified as:

- needles used in a patient's vein or artery
- deep injury
- visible contamination of the device with blood
- late-stage disease in the source patient.

It is essential that every effort is made to prevent needlestick injuries as many organisms are potentially transmissible in the occupational setting via percutaneous (sharp) or mucocutaneous (mucous membrane/broken skin) routes. The Health Protection Agency suggest that 38% of incidents reported to them could have been prevented if procedures related to safe handling and disposal of sharps and clinical waste had been adhered to (Health Protection Agency 2005b).

RISK MANAGEMENT

Healthcare will always involve a degree of potential risk, but it is important to minimise that risk whenever practicable. A number of incidents are the consequence of poor working practices often due to inadequate training or facilities, or environmental issues. Clinical governance provides a framework within which healthcare organisations can work to improve and assure the quality of clinical services for patients (National Health

Service Executive 1999). By focusing on the activities involved in the delivery of high quality care to patients, it allows for the production and agreement of risk assessments that will support and guide staff whilst controlling risk.

There are three main elements:

1. setting clear quality standards
2. ensuring local delivery
3. monitoring delivery.

Clinical governance seeks to remedy deficiency in a service. This can be addressed by enhancing the skills of existing staff through training or professional development and by developing new staff with a set of skills and competencies to fit the new circumstances. It is important to have the right number of people with the right skills.

Good information is an essential feature of quality; this includes:

- identifying the scope for improvement
- monitoring progress to see if planned development or investment has resulted in the desired change
- comparing with local services and counterparts
- monitoring adverse outcome of care

This will ensure clinical governance can detect and analyse from experience, including adverse events and service failures, so that we learn to improve activities (Health Protection Agency 2005b).

The key to clinical governance is risk management using a system of continuous risk assessment and prioritisation and establishing a comprehensive risk register. The aim is to achieve optimum balance between quality care and the provision of services which are safe, by a continuous cycle of identification, assessment, control, monitoring and review of risk. All healthcare workers must be aware of the risk assessments in their area of work and work activities and the relevant procedures or control measures to be adopted to reduce identified risk. To achieve optimum risk management, healthcare workers have a responsibility to make full and proper use of any equipment and systems of work provided for them and attend any training appropriate to their work.

Risk assessments must be suitable, sufficient and show that a proper check has been made – checking who and how many may be affected, dealing with the significant hazards and evaluating if the precautions required are reasonable so that the risk remains low.

The Health and Safety Executive (2004a) identified five steps to risk assessment (Box 6.2).

Hazards to healthcare workers related to cannulation and venepuncture include:

- chemicals – e.g. chlorhexidine in alcohol, which is inflammable
- blood and body fluids – e.g. needlestick injury, contamination of mucous membranes
- absence of needle-free and needle-safe systems
- absence of personal protective equipment (PPE) – e.g. gloves
- allergy to equipment – e.g. latex gloves
- height of work – back strain
- poor light – eye strain
- poor disposal of sharps – e.g. needles in rubbish bag.

Hazards to patients include:

- bleeding, bruising – inexperienced worker
- allergy to equipment use – e.g. dressing, latex
- infection – e.g. poor technique, non-sterile equipment
- chemicals – e.g. chlorhexidine in alcohol, which is inflammable.

More control measures may be required if, for example:

1. practice does not meet legal standards and recognised good practice, i.e. Control of Substances Hazardous to Health (COSHH), PPE
2. adequate information and training is not provided.

See Examples 1 and 2 of risk assessments in Box 6.2.

Box 6.2 Risk assessment

Five Steps to Risk Assessment

- Step One – Look for hazards (anything that can cause harm).
- Step Two – Decide who might be harmed and how.
- Step Three – Evaluate the risk and decide whether the existing precautions are adequate or whether more should be done (chance that someone will be harmed, can it be removed, if not, how it can be controlled).
- Step Four – Record your findings.
- Step Five – Review your assessment and revise it if necessary. A date should be set for review; at this time new hazards may be found that require new assessments being produced.

Example 1: Risk assessment for venepuncture

| Department: Ward 8C | TASK/ACTIVITY: Venepuncture | | REFERENCE NUMBER: 1010 | | | | |

DESCRIPTION OF RISKS (What ifs)	CAUSAL FACTORS	RISK CONTROL MEASURES IN PLACE	L	S	RR	ACTION PLAN TO REDUCE RISK
Healthcare worker develops HIV following needlestick injury to staff	1. Needlestick injury 2. Failure of HIV prophylaxis to prevent seroconversion 3. Poor compliance to PPE 4. Poor technique	a. Occupational health service b. Accident policy c. COSHH/PPE policy d. HIV policy e. Post-exposure prophylaxis policy f. Prophylactic drugs available g. Sharps policy h. Waste policy i. Orientation and mandatory training programmes	1	3	Low	1. Implement needle-less systems 2. Continue education and training 3. Increase supervision

Example 2: Risk assessment for cannulation

Department: Ward 8 C	TASK/ACTIVITY: Cannulation					REFERENCE NUMBER: 1011	
DESCRIPTION OF RISKS (What ifs)	CAUSAL FACTORS	RISK CONTROL MEASURES IN PLACE	L	S	RR		ACTION PLAN TO REDUCE RISK
Patient's cannula site becomes infected leading to septicaemia	1. Breach in aseptic technique 2. Nonsterile equipment 3. Inadequate skin cleansing 4. Inadequate hand cleansing 5. Translocation of microorganisms from another body site 6. Cannula left in situ too long	a. Cannulation policy b. COSHH/PPE policy c. Aseptic technique procedure. d. Antibiotic policy e. Observation policy f. Waste policy g. Orientation and mandatory training programmes.	1	3	Mod.		1. Continue education and training 2. Increase supervision

Key to codes:

Rating Score 1–5 **(for both Likelihood and Significance)**

L: Likelihood of risk occurring
S: Significance of risk if it does occur
RR: Risk Rating (of risk)

1: Insignificant
2: Minor
3: Moderate
4: Major
5: Catastrophic

Specimen handling and transportation

Care must be taken when obtaining diagnostic specimens. This includes:

- protection of the healthcare worker from the blood and body fluids that may be generated by the specimen collection
- protection for the patient from acquiring an infection during the specimen collection
- protection of the environment by ensuring spillage does not occur.

Labelling of specimens and specimen request cards

Specimens must be correctly labelled with the following details:

- **Patient details**: first name, surname, hospital number, ward or doctor surgery details, date of birth.
- **Source of specimen**: intravenous device or vein.
- **Type of specimen**: venous blood sample.
- **Type of test with reason for request:** i.e. blood culture for suspected infection.
- **Time and date of collection**.
- **Signature.**
- **Specimens posing a risk of infection**: if a patient is known to have an infection such as HIV, hepatitis B or C, the specimen request card and the specimen container must be labelled with a biohazard sticker.
- **Other potential problems**: for example, with a specimen obtained following an injection of a diagnostic dose of radioactivity the specimen should be labelled with a radioactive warning sticker.

Specimen containers

Specimen containers must be sufficiently strong and leakproof to comply with the British Standard BS ISO 6710:1995.

Specimen transport bags

After labelling, all specimens must be placed in an individual transparent plastic transport bag and sealed. The request card must not be placed in the bag with the specimen; a separate pocket for the request card should be an integral part of the specimen transport bag (Health and Safety Executive 2003). If a specimen container does break or leak, the blood will be contained within the plastic transport bag. By keeping the request card separate from the specimen, if there is a leak, the request card will not become contaminated.

On-site transportation of specimens

Carrying boxes
All specimens must be transported in a carrier box with a lid, made of a smooth impervious material such as plastic or metal, which will retain liquid if the specimen leaks and can be easily disinfected and cleaned (Health and Safety Executive 2003).

Pneumatic air tube systems
Pneumatic air tube transport system provide an efficient, rapid and safe means of sending specimens from their place of origin to the laboratories.

Local policies must be followed as it is important that specimen are carefully handled so they do not become damaged and leak. Contamination of the tube is prevented by staff who are properly trained in its use and by using suitable specimen containers for the pneumatic air tube containers being used.

Carriage by post
Specimens other than hazard group 4 specimens that have been correctly labelled and bagged can be packed in packaging that complies with the Royal Mail packaging specifications and sent by the normal post. Hazard group 4 includes biological agents that cause severe human disease and are a serious hazard to employees; an example is viral haemorrhagic fever – see Box 6.3 (Health and Safety Executive 2003).

Carriage by road
The carriage of dangerous goods and use of transportable pressure equipment regulations (Health and Safety Executive 2004b) include diagnostic specimens within hazard groups 1, 2 and 3

> **Box 6.3 Definition of hazard groups**
>
> Hazard group 1: Biological agent unlikely to cause human disease.
> Hazard group 2: Biological agent that can cause human disease but is unlikely
> to spread in the community and there is usually effective prophylaxis or
> effective treatment available.
> Hazard group 3: Biological agent that can cause serious human disease.
> Presents a hazard to employees, may spread in the community, usually
> effective prophylaxis and effective treatment available.
> Hazard group 4: Biological agent that causes serious human disease, serious
> hazard to employees, can spread in community, usually no effective
> prophylaxis or treatment.

(see Box 6.3). The general requirements within these regulations require staff responsible for such carriage to be appropriately trained, and the specimens to be appropriately boxed and labelled, with appropriate documentation included with each consignment. Emergency equipment and procedures to be followed must be available in the event of accidents. This means that every effort has been made to ensure that specimens are transported appropriately and safely but if an accident does occur the environment will not become contaminated and those helping to deal with the accident will be aware of the potential risk from the specimens (Health and Safety Executive 2004b).

CONCLUSION

Healthcare organisations must have systems in place to ensure:

- risk of infection to patients and staff is minimised
- risks associated with the acquisition and use of medical devices are minimised
- as far as reasonably practicable, all reusable medical devices are properly decontaminated prior to use (Department of Health 2004).

This chapter has provided infection control and risk assessment information related to venepuncture and cannulation. The information is designed to ensure that the reader is aware of what is involved in achieving good practice which if adopted will reduce the risk to themselves and their patients.

REFERENCES

Ayliffe, G.A.J., Fraise, A.P., Geddes, A.M. & Mitchell, K. (2002) *Control of Hospital Infection. A Practical Handbook*, 4th edn. Arnold, London.

Blaivas, M. &Lyon, M. (2006) The effect of ultrasound guidance on the perceived difficulty of emergency nurse-obtained peripheral IV access. *Journal of Emergency Medicine*, **31**(4), 407–410.

British Committee for Standards in Haematology (BCSH) (1999) Guidelines for the administration of blood and blood components and the management of transfused patients. *Transfusion Medicine*, **9**, 227–239.

Calfee, D.P. & Farr, B.M. (2002) Comparison of four antiseptic preparations for skin in the prevention of contamination of percutaneously drawn blood cultures: a randomised trial. *Journal of Clinical Microbiology*, **40**(5), 1660–1665.

CDC – Centers for Disease Control and Prevention 2002 Guidelines for the prevention of intravascular catheter-related infections. *MMWR – Morbidity and Mortality Weekly Report*, **51**, RR10.

Christiaens, G., Barbier, C. & Mustsers, J, *et al.* (2006) Hand hygiene: first measures to control nosocomial infection. *Revue Medical de Liege*, **61**(1), 31–36.

Collignon, P. (1994) Intravenous catheter associated sepsis: a common problem. An Australian study of intravenous catheter associated sepsis. *Medical Journal of Australia*, **161**(6), 374–378.

Department of Health (2001) Standard principles for preventing hospital acquired infections. *Journal of Hospital Infection*, **47**(Suppl.), S21–S37.

Department of Health (2003a) *Winning Ways. Working Together to reduce Healthcare Associated Infection in England*. Department of Health Publications, London.

Department of Health (2003b) *A Matron's Charter: An Action Plan for Cleaner Hospitals*. Department of Health, London.

Department of Health (2004) *HIV post-exposure prophylaxis. Guidance from the UK Chief Medical Officer*. Department of Health, London.

Department of Health (2007a) *Saving Lives: Reducing Infection, Delivering Clean and Safe Care. High Impact interventions No 2. Peripheral Intravenous Cannula Care Bundle*. Department of Health, London.

Department of Health (2007b) *Saving Lives: Reducing Infection, Delivering Clean and Safe Care. High Impact Interventions. Taking Blood Cultures*. Department of Health, London.

Department of Health (2008) *Clean Safe Care. Reducing Infection and Saving Lives*. Department of Health, London.

Dietze, B., Rath, A., Wendt, C. & Martiny, H. (2001) Survival of MRSA on sterile goods packaging. *Journal of Hospital Infection*, **49**(4), 255–274.

Dougherty, L. & Watson, J. (2008) Vascular access devices. In: *The Royal Marsden Hospital Manual of Clinical Nursing Procedures* (eds L. Dougherty & S. Lister), 7th edn, pp. 856–918. Wiley Blackwell, Oxford.

Eggimann, P., Sax, H. & Pittet, D. (2004) Catheter related infections. *Microbes and Infection*, **6**(11), 1033–1042.

Gabriel, J. (2006) Vascular access. In: *Nursing in Haematological Oncology* (ed. M. Grundy), 2nd edn, pp. 295–320. Baillière Tindall, Edinburgh.

Gordin, F.M., Schultz, M.E., Huber, R.A. & Gill, J.A. (2005) Reduction in nosocomial transmission of drug resistant bacteria after introduction of an alcohol-based handrub. *Infection Control and Hospital Epidemiology*, **26**(7)650–653.

Hadaway, L.C. (2003) Skin flora and infection. *Journal of Infusion Nursing*, **26**(1), 44–48.

Hart, S. (2006) Prevention of infection. In: *Nursing in Haematological Oncology* (ed. M. Grundy), 2nd edn, pp. 321–338. Baillière Tindall, Edinburgh.

Hart, S. (2007) Using an aseptic technique in reducing the risk of infection. *Nursing Standard*, **21**(47), 43–48.

Health and Safety Executive (2003) *Safe Working and the Prevention of Infection in Clinical Laboratories and Similar Facilities*. HSE Books.

Health and Safety Executive (2004a) *Five Steps to Risk Assessment*. Health and Safety Executive.

Health and Safety Executive (2004b) *Carriage of Dangerous Goods and Use of Transportable Pressure Equipment Regulations* 2004 (the Carriage Regulations). Health and Safety Executive.

Health Protection Agency (2005a) *Occupational transmission of HIV*. Health Protection Agency.

Health Protection Agency (2005b) *Eye of the Needle*. Health Protection Agency.

Jeanes, A. (2005) Keeping hospital clean: how nurses can reduce healthcare associated infection. *Professional Nurse* **20**(6), 35–37.

Kampf, G. & Kramer, A. (2004) Epidemiologic background of hand hygiene and evaluation of the most important agents for scrubs and rubs. *Clinical Microbiology Reviews*, **17**(4), 863–893.

Kjonniksen, I., Andersen, B.M., Sondenaa, V.G. & Segadal, L. (2002) Preoperative hair removal-a systematic literature review. *AORN J*, **75**(5), 928–938.

Maki, D.G., Ringer, M. & Alvarado, C.J. (1991) Prospective randomised trial of povidone-iodine, alcohol and chlorhexidine for prevention of infection associated with central venous and arterial catheters. *Lancet* **338**(8763)339-343.

Marini, M.A., Giangregorio, M. & Kraskinski, J.C. (2004) Complying with the occupational safety and health administration's blood borne pathogen standard: implementing needleless systems and intravenous safety devices. *Pediatric Emergency Care*, **20**(3), 209–214.

McLaws, M.L. & Taylor, P.C. (2003) The Hospital Infection Standardised Surveillance (HISS) programme: analysis of a two year pilot. *Journal of Hospital Infection*, **53**(4), 374–378.

McParland, J., Scott, P.A., Arndt, M, *et al.* (2000) Autonomy and clinical practice. 3: Issues of patient consent. *British Journal of Nursing*, **9**(10), 660–665.

National Health Service Estates (2002) *Infection Control in the Built Environment*. Department of Health.

National Health Service Estates (2003) *A Guide to the Decontamination of Reusable Surgical Instruments*. Department of Health.

National Health Service Executive (1999) *Clinical Governance: Quality in the New NHS*. Department of Health, London.

Niel-Weise, B.S., Wille, J.C. & van den Brock, P.J. (2005) Hair removal policies in clean surgery: systematic review of randomized, controlled trials. *Infection Control and Hospital Epidemiology*, **26**(12), 923–928.

Pratt, R.J., Pellowe, C.M., Wilson, J.A., *et al.* (2007) Epic2: National evidence-based guidelines for preventing healthcare-associated infections in NHS hospitals in England. *Journal of Hospital Infection*, **65**(Suppl. 1), S1–64.

Preston, R.M. (2005) Aseptic technique: evidence-based approach for patient safety. *British Journal of Nursing*, **14**(10), 540–542.

Royal College of Nursing (RCN) (2005a) *Good Practice in Infection Prevention and Control. Guidance for Nursing Staff*. RCN, London.

Royal College of Nursing (RCN) (2005b) *Competencies: An Education and Training Competency Framework for Capillary Blood Sampling and Venepuncture in Children and Young People*. RCN, London.

Scott, P.A., Valimak, M., Leino-Kilpi, H., *et al.* (2003) Autonomy, privacy and informed consent 1:concepts and definitions. *British Journal of Nursing*, **12**(1), 43–47.

Sexton, T., Clarke, P., O'Neill, E., *et al.* (2006) Environmental reservoirs of methicillin resistant *Staphylococcus aureus* in isolation rooms: correlation with patient isolates and implications for hospital hygiene. *Journal of Hospital Infection*, **62**(2), 187–194.

Sickbert-Bennett, E.E., Weber, D.J., Gergen-Teague, M.F., *et al.* (2005) Comparative efficacy of hand hygiene agents in the reduction of bacteria and viruses. *American Journal of Infection Control*, **33**(2), 67–77.

Taylor, K., Plowman, R. & Roberts, J.A. (2001) *The Challenge of Hospital Acquired Infection*. National Audit Office.

Tripepi-Bova, K.A., Woods, K.D. & Loach, M.C. (1997) A comparison of transparent polyurethane and dry gauze dressings for peripheral i.v. catheter sites: rates of phlebitis, infiltration, and dislodgment by patients. *American Journal of Critical Care*, **6**(5), 377–381.

Vincent, J.L., Bihari, D.J., Suter, P.M., *et al.* (1995) The prevalence of nosocomial infection in intensive care units in Europe. Results of the European prevalence of infection in intensive care (EPIC) study. EPIC international advisory committee. *JAMA*, **274**(8), 639–644.

Warren, D.K., Zack, J.E., Cox, M., *et al.* (2003) An educational intervention to prevent catheter-associated bloodstream infections in a nonteaching, community medicine center. *Critical Care Medicine*, **31**(7), 1959–1963.

Procedures for Venepuncture and Cannulation

7

Annie de Verteuil

LEARNING OUTCOMES

The practitioner will be able to:

❏ Describe how to prepare the patient and environment for the procedures.

❏ Explain the techniques applied for the procedures.

❏ Identify equipment required for the procedure of venepuncture/cannulation.

❏ Demonstrate how to correctly carry out the procedure for venepuncture/cannulation.

INTRODUCTION

The aim of this chapter is to provide the practitioner with an overview of the procedures for performing both venepuncture and cannulation. The technique used by the practitioner is essential to achieving a successful venepuncture or cannulation. The practitioner will be guided in relation to preparation of the patient and the environment; both of which are important initial steps. The equipment required and rationale for each of the

Venepuncture and Cannulation, first edition. Edited by Sarah Phillips, Mary Collins and Lisa Dougherty. Published 2011 by Blackwell Publishing Ltd. © 2011 Blackwell Publishing Ltd.

steps required for both procedures is presented. However, each time these procedures are performed there is the potential to encounter problems, and troubleshooting for some of the more common problems is also considered in this chapter.

PREPARATION OF THE ENVIRONMENT AND THE PRACTITIONER

Adequate preparation of the environment is essential if either of these procedures are to be performed proficiently and the practitioner will need to carry out a risk assessment of the area in which they intend to undertake the procedure.

Lighting

The support of adequate lighting is essential to assist visual inspection of the patient's veins and will increase a successful outcome (Weinstein 2007). Good lighting is also important to enhance the safety of the practitioner when disposing of sharps after the procedure has taken place. The practitioner may need to consider an extra bedside light or flashlight to assist visibility if necessary (Perucca 2010).

Temperature

A patient's veins are sensitive to temperature and vasoconstriction may occur if the patient is cold or anxious. Therefore, the environment where the procedure is to be undertaken needs to be a warm and comfortable temperature, which will enhance the patient's venous access. However, if the room is too hot it may result in the patient feeling faint.

Privacy

When considering the environment, a private area to perform the procedure will ensure that the practitioner is not distracted or interrupted. Patient privacy can be achieved either by screening off the area where the procedure is to be performed, or by using a separate room. If the patient has visitors, the patient may prefer that the visitors are asked to wait elsewhere during the process, or they may welcome the support of someone they know who can act as a distraction during the procedure. Patients should therefore be asked as to their preference (Dougherty 2008).

Positioning of the practitioner

When preparing the environment the practitioner needs to consider their own personal comfort. This may require them to raise or lower the bed to the appropriate height or provide themselves with a chair or stool to reduce any unnecessary stretching and bending during the process (Dougherty 2008). If the procedure is being undertaken in an alternative care setting the above consideration should always be taken into account (Perucca 2010). The equipment being used during the procedure should always be in close proximity to the practitioner, with particular care being taken around the positioning of the sharps disposal container which should remain within arm's reach during the process.

Equipment

The practitioner needs to be adequately prepared by assembling all the necessary equipment required to perform the procedure and make sure they have sufficient supplies in order to complete the task. This will avoid unnecessary interruptions during the process. It is essential that they have a range of cannulae or needles in various gauge sizes to undertake each procedure assembled in a receiver, tray or onto a clean trolley, to transport to the patient. The equipment needs to be sterile and for single use only (MDA 2001). The packaging needs to be examined to make sure it has not been damaged and thus possibly contaminated (Dougherty 2008). The expiry dates on all equipment, packaging and blood bottles should be checked. When the practitioner is ready to perform venepuncture the required bottles need to be assembled in close proximity to the patient and within the practitioner's visual field.

Sharps and waste disposal

An important aspect of safe sharps disposal is the positioning of the sharps disposal container, which needs to be in arm's reach of the procedure to enable safe and immediate disposal of the sharp and reduce the risk of the practitioner receiving a needlestick injury (Health Protection Agency 2005). The practitioner must always personally dispose of any sharps used into a sharps container. This container should be rigid, puncture resistant, disposable, and leakproof with a lockable lid. Care should be taken not to overfill the recommended level. It should then be disposed of in accordance with current guidance (Pellowe *et al.* 2007).

Preparation of the patient

The patient's comfort and safety must be considered, as potentially any patient may be subject to the unpleasant sensation of feeling faint or even experiencing a vasovagal episode during the process. The patient should be positioned on a bed, chair or couch which has a back rest that will enable the patient to be positioned flat in the event that the patient feels faint (Black & Hughes 1997). The patient's arm should be supported so that he or she is able to keep their arm straight during the process, which can be achieved by supporting the selected limb with a pillow (Perucca 2010). It is important to explain to the patient why it is necessary to keep the arm straight when taking blood from the antecubital veins. A straight arm will assist the practitioner when palpating the veins at the outset and any movement may stop the blood from flowing freely into the blood collection system.

It is also important that the patient is adequately prepared both psychologically and physically. A calm and confident approach will relax the patient and facilitate compliance (Weinstein 2007). The practitioner needs to discuss and explore the patient's previous knowledge of undergoing the process, and ensure they provide a thorough explanation of what should be expected and may be experienced when undergoing either procedure (Dougherty 2008). For further information see Chapter 10.

TECHNIQUES REQUIRED TO PERFORM VENEPUNCTURE

(For selection of the vein see Chapter 5 and for preparation of the skin see Chapter 6.)

Once the practitioner is ready to perform the procedure the vein will need to be stabilised using the non-dominant hand just below the insertion site. This is known as 'anchoring'. The traction needs to be applied as soon as the practitioner is ready to advance the needle as anchoring the skin will provide the counter tension essential to ensure smooth entry of the needle when the bevel is in the uppermost position (Perucca 2010; Springhouse 2002). Using the fingers of the anchoring hand to support the elbow helps to prevent the apprehensive patient moving their arm as the needle is inserted (McCall & Tankersley 2008). When the veins are visible and palpable the practitioner can insert the needle directly into the vein. When the practitioner encounters smaller veins, the indirect method may be adopted. This is when the needle is inserted into the skin and then the smaller vein is relocated and the needle advanced into the vein, enabling a more gentle entry for delicate veins (McCall & Tankersley 2008). On no account should the practitioner have more than two attempts (Lavery & Ingram 2005). Each attempt will result in an increase in the patient's perception of pain experienced. Each attempt will result in a risk of infection with increased entry sites.

Equipment required to perform venepuncture

- Clinically clean tray or receiver
- Disposable tourniquet
- Chlorhexidine in 70% alcohol impregnated swabs
- Vacuumed specimen collection bottles
- Appropriate needles or winged infusion devices
- Sterile cotton wool or gauze
- Tape or adhesive plaster
- Closed blood collection system holder
- Clinically clean gloves
- Sharps bin
- Specimen request form

Venepuncture procedure

At the outset the practitioner will need to consider all of the above-mentioned environmental issues and appropriate preparation of the patient before performing venepuncture.

Step	Action	Rationale
Preparation		
1	Prepare the area by considering the lighting, privacy, local temperature and preparation of equipment to be used.	To ensure that the patient as well as the practitioner are adequately prepared.
2	Position patient on a chair or couch.	To maintain safety of patient if they experience vasovagal faint. Also for the patient's comfort.
3	Approach the patient in a confident manner and check identity of patient either by checking request slip against patient's details on wrist-band or by the patient verbally confirming full name and date of birth.	To reduce the patient's anxiety and alleviate the potential of causing vasoconstriction of the vein. To ensure that the sample is being obtained from the correct patient (NPSA 2006).
4	Give a thorough explanation of the procedure, allowing time for the patient to ask any questions and discuss any previous difficulties that may have arisen.	To obtain consent and in discussing patient's previous history consider the most appropriate equipment to perform the procedure effectively (Lavery 2003).

5	Position patient's arm by supporting on a pillow.	To maintain patient's comfort during the procedure.
6	Collect sufficient quantities of all necessary equipment for venepuncture (see list above).	To avoid any unnecessary interruptions during the procedure.
7	Ensure that packaging has been checked with seals intact and that the equipment has not expired. Take all equipment to the patient.	To prevent the use of bottles with no vacuum and to avoid the risk of using faulty or contaminated equipment.
8	Perform effective hand washing technique using soap and water or appropriate alcohol rub.	To minimise the risk of infection and maintain asepsis (Franklin 1999; Hindley 2004).
9	Cover any visibly broken skin with a suitable waterproof dressing.	To reduce the risk of contamination by blood to the practitioner.

Site assessment and selection

| 10 | Apply tourniquet 7–8 cm above desired location. | To create adequate venous filling (RCN 2010). |
| 11 | Assess the patient's veins. | To verify the most suitable vein to access. |

12	To assist venous filling, the patient can (a) Clench fist then relax, repeat this action several times. (b) Hold the arm straight with the palm of the hand facing upwards. (c) Immerse the limb into a bowl of hot water.	To aid venous filling and increase the prominence of a patient's veins in order to ascertain the direction of the veins pathway and its depth and identify any surrounding structures that need to be avoided, tendons and arteries.
13	Release the tourniquet.	To maintain patient's comfort. Minimise the effect of the reduced blood flow on the specimen composition (McCall & Tankersley 2008).
14	Position all the required assembled equipment within practitioner's visual field, on the non-dominant side to enable easy selection of equipment.	To reduce any unnecessary movement of the practitioner during the procedure.
15	Select the appropriate size needle and type of device and assemble the equipment.	To reduce trauma or damage to the vein.
16	Wash hands with antibacterial soap and water and dry or use antibacterial alcohol hand gel.	To minimise the risk of infection (DH 2005).

17	Reapply tourniquet.	To create adequate venous filling and to increase prominence of veins by obstructing venous return.
18	Put on gloves.	To minimise the practitioner's risk of contamination by blood (ICNA 2003; DH 2007).
19	Clean the chosen site with an appropriate cleaning solution for 30 seconds using sufficient pressure to remove surface dirt and debris, and allow the skin to air dry for a further 30 seconds.	To reduce the risk of contamination.
20	Do not re-palpate the skin after cleaning has occurred or contaminate by fanning with hand or swab.	To maintain asepsis.

Insertion

a. **Using a NEEDLE AND HOLDER (for winged infusion device go to b)**

| 21a | Apply traction with the thumb or forefinger onto the skin a few centimetres below the proposed insertion site. | To immobilise the vein and ensure adequate counter tension to facilitate ease of entry for the needle. |

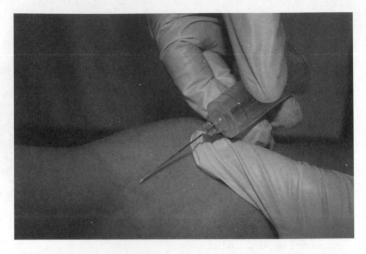

Fig. 7.1 Correct hold of needle holder. Used with permission of Vein Train Ltd.

22a   Pick up assembled needle and holder in the dominant hand with the middle and index finger on the underside of the holder, and the thumb gripping the holder on the upper side (see Fig. 7.1).

To maintain grip on the holder and to prevent any obstruction of access when attaching the blood bottles.

23a   Inspect needle and ensure bevel of needle is facing upwards (see Fig. 7.2).

To assist practitioner in delivering successful smooth pain-free access to vein.

24a   Insert the needle at an angle of approximately 15–30 degrees depending on the location and size of the vein (see Figs 7.3 and 7.4).

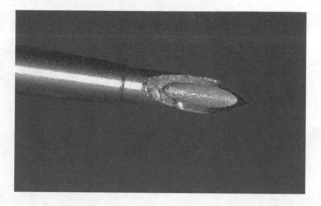

Fig. 7.2 Bevel of needle uppermost (in vein). Used with permission of Vein Train Ltd.

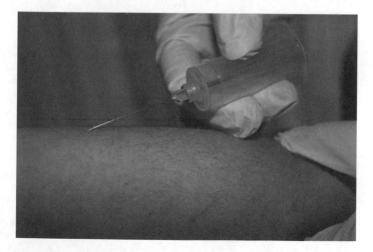

Fig. 7.3 Illustration of shallow angle of insertion – 15 degrees (needle and holder). Used with permission of Vein Train Ltd.

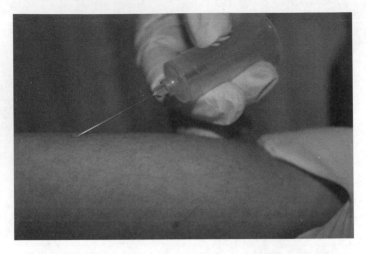

Fig. 7.4 Illustration of deeper angle of insertion – 30 degrees (needle and holder). Used with permission of Vein Train Ltd.

25a   Advance the needle approximately 1–2 mm into the vein maintaining the hold described in action 22a, allowing the middle finger and index finger on the underside of the holder to rest against the patient's skin (Fig. 7.1).

To prevent the needle advancing too far and causing damage to the intima of the vein and to maintain a steady grip on the holder, ensuring that it does not penetrate too far into the vein causing a through puncture (which could result in haematoma formation).

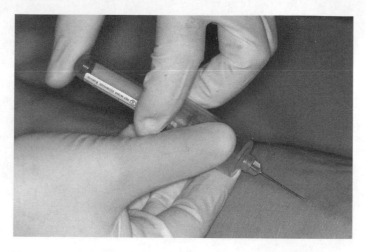

Fig. 7.5 Push bottle in using wings of holder and thumb on bottle end.

26a Maintain anchoring described in action 21a.

(a) Attach the blood bottles in the recommended order of draw into the holder.

(b) With the non-dominant hand using the third finger and index finger directly above the ears/wings of the holder.

(c) Use the thumb to push against the base of the blood bottle as it penetrates the rubber sleeve that covers the needle as shown in Fig. 7.5.

(a) To prevent any transference of additives from one bottle to another.

(b) To maintain a steadfast grip on the holder when penetrating the rubber cap on the blood sample bottle with the multi-sample needle, and enable the vacuum in the bottle to draw the blood from the patient's vein.

(c) To support and steady the blood collection bottle, and ensure that the vacuum is functioning.

143

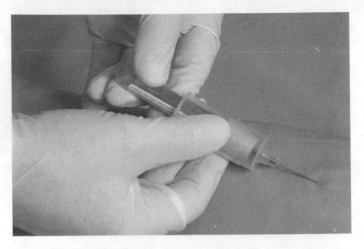

Fig. 7.6 Rotating bottle to view correct fill amount.

27a   Attach the blood bottle onto the vacuumed collection system. Ensure that the label appears on the underside of the bottle by turning the bottle clockwise or anti-clockwise as the blood fills the bottle (see Fig. 7.6).

To ensure that the practitioner has good visibility of the filling of the bottle to check it is filled to the appropriate level.

b.   **Using a WINGED INFUSION DEVICE (for needle and holder go to a)**

Used for collecting blood on infants and children and difficult or hand veins of adults.

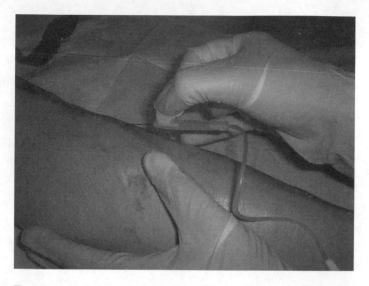

Fig. 7.7 Holding wings correctly of winged blood collection set. Used with permission of Vein Train Ltd.

21b	Assemble winged infusion device and grip the wings in the dominant hand between the thumb and index finger with the bevel of needle facing upwards (Fig. 7.7).	To assist practitioner in delivering successful smooth pain-free access to vein.
22b	Access the selected vein with a shallow angle of entry at an approximate angle of 5–15 degrees depending on the location and size of the vein and advance the needle approximately 1 mm into the vein.	To prevent the needle advancing too far and causing damage to the intima of the vein or a through puncture; this could result in a haematoma formation.

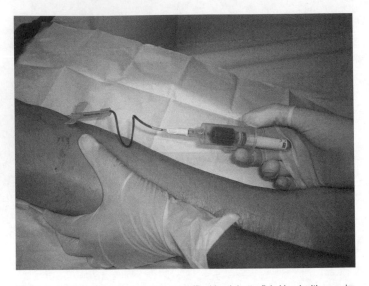

Fig. 7.8 Blood in tubing upon vein entry (flashback butterfly). Used with permission of Vein Train Ltd.

23b	Observe for blood in the tubing (Fig. 7.8) then attach blood bottles (Fig. 7.9).	To verify that the needle has entered the lumen of the vein.
28	Once the bottle has filled, remove and insert next bottle until all samples taken.	To ensure correct volume of blood taken and all required samples are taken.

Needle removal and site care

29	Release tourniquet.	To decrease pressure within the vein.

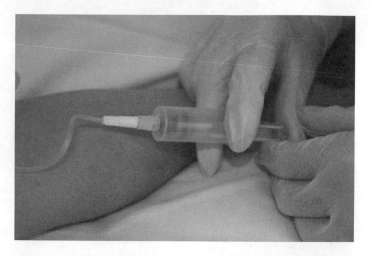

Fig. 7.9 Push bottle in using wings of holder and thumb (butterfly). Used with permission of Vein Train Ltd.

| 30 | Maintain anchoring, and remove the last blood collection bottle with the non-dominant hand, grip the bottle with thumb and middle finger and use the index finger to push the bottle away from the holder on the underside of the wings. | To ensure that the needle does not penetrate further into the vein. |

147

| 31 | Place a sterile swab over the puncture site, and only apply pressure once the needle has been fully withdrawn.
When possible request the patient to apply pressure on the site whilst keeping the arm fully extended. This should exceed 1 minute if the patient is on anticoagulants or is on thrombocytopenic therapy. | To prevent pain on removal of needle.
To prevent leakage, preserve vein and avoid haematoma.
To prevent bruising (McCall & Tankersley 2008). |

Disposal and transportation

32	Activate safety guard if appropriate and then discard needle and holder as a single unit immediately into the sharps bin.	To reduce risk of needlestick injury.
33	Gently invert the bottles as per manufacturer's instructions.	To ensure correct adequate mixing of blood specimen and additive. To negate the need for further unnecessary blood tests.
34	Remove gloves and dispose in appropriate clinical waste area.	To prevent cross-contamination.

35	Label bottles carefully in the patient's presence and as per local policy and NBS policy (NBS 2007).	To check and ensure that the blood results relate to the correct patient, and details are clear and legible to the laboratory. In the case of pre-transfusion testing, if there is mismatch between the form and the bottle, the laboratory staff must not process the sample until identification is confirmed, even if this may lead to a delay in treatment for patients or a retest (NBS 2008).
36	Ensure appropriate labelling is carried out e.g. to indicate an infection risk.	To comply with universal precautions.
37	Inspect the puncture site and if bleeding has discontinued cover with an appropriate dressing.	To ensure there is no further bleeding. To check that the puncture site is covered with a suitable dressing, having ascertained the patient has no allergy to chosen dressing.
38	Dispose of other clinical waste.	To prevent cross-contamination.
39	Review the patient's comfort.	To ensure that the patient does not require any further intervention before the practitioner departs.

| 40 | Follow hospital procedure for collection and transportation to the laboratory. | To ensure swift collection of urgent requests and prompt results. |

Troubleshooting

If blood stops flowing after initial flashback
The practitioner should consider the following:

Cause	Prevention	Action
Needle may have penetrated through the vein (Fig. 7.10).	Angle of entry may have been too steep. Practitioner needs to acknowledge the distance between the needle holder and the entry site.	Withdraw needle slightly to encourage blood withdrawal; however, if bruising is evident needle needs to be fully withdrawn and pressure applied to puncture point.
Needle may be in contact with a valve.	Palpation to identify location of valve.	Withdraw the needle slightly to move it from the valve.

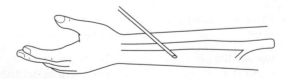

Fig. 7.10 Through puncture – needle punctured through both walls of vein. Used with permission of Vein Train Ltd.

Venous spasm as a result of mechanical irritation		This can be resolved in some cases by simply removing and reapplying the blood bottle, or simply massaging the vein above point of entry. Consider attaching a syringe to the winged blood collection system to reduce vacuum.
Vein too small	Avoid where possible, reassess or relocate to a different site. Better vein selection.	Consider the use of different collecting system. Smaller gauge needles. Winged blood collection system can be angled much closer to the skin and when attached to a syringe can reduce the vacuum on the vein as the blood is expelled.
Vein collapsed	Tourniquet too tight. Vacuum too vigorous.	Allow veins to refill by releasing and then reapplying the tourniquet.
Poor technique when handling equipment	Bevel of needle may be occluding blood flow by adhering to the vein wall.	Turn the needle and holder in a clockwise or anti-clockwise direction to release the bevel from the wall of the vein. Winged infusion devices need to be tilted gently in an upward direction to alter the angle of the bevel and enhance the flow of blood.

Faulty equipment, e.g. loss of vacuum in blood collection bottles.	Always check the expiry date on the blood collection bottles; if they are out of date the vacuum may not be effective.	Take extra blood collection bottles to patient to attach in case there are problems with equipment.

If on entry blood is observed to leak around the needle
The practitioner should consider the following:

Cause	**Prevention**	**Action**
Practitioner advances needle slowly and bevel contacts vein before fully under skin.	Raise awareness of this outcome when supervising. Tourniquet may be too tight.	Confident approach when inserting needle. Explain reason to the patient.

TECHNIQUES TO PERFORM CANNULATION

There are two methods for inserting a cannula – the direct or indirect method – and choice will depend on the practitioner's assessment of the patient's veins. The indirect method of approach is more suitable for smaller fragile veins. The cannula is inserted into the skin and the vein is relocated before the cannula is gently advanced into the vein. When the vein is situated in deeper subcutaneous tissue and is not as visible, the practitioner can utilise palpation to locate (Perucca 2010). The practitioner would then insert the cannula choosing a direct method of insertion.

There are also a number of methods when anchoring the vein prior to cannulation. The vein can be stabilised using the thumb to stretch the skin in a downward direction below the proposed insertion site (McCall & Tankersley 2008). This is more suitable if the vein is situated in the deeper skin tissue and the approach angle of the needle needs to be steeper. If the patient's veins are more superficial, the technique for stabilising the vein would be to stretch it between the forefinger and thumb. Alternatively the practitioner can place a hand under the patient's arm whilst applying traction with the thumb and forefinger on either side of the vein. This will create an even traction, and is particularly effective in older patients whose skin lacks collagen, subcutaneous fat and the ability to stay fully hydrated (McCall & Tankersley 2008).

The angle and grip that the practitioner adopts when the needle approaches the entry site will be influenced by the depth of the vein in the subcutaneous tissue. For example, some cannulae have finger guards to stabilise the cannula as it is advanced into the vein. When the cannulation needle (stylet) has been inserted into the chosen vein, the blood will flow into the chamber of the cannula, indicating that entry into the vein has been successful. This is acknowledged as first 'flashback'; however, if the posterior wall of the vein is punctured the 'flashback' will stop. If using a smaller gauge cannula it may take slightly longer for the blood to fill the chamber (Perucca 2010). With every cannula insertion once the flashback of blood has been acknowledged, the practitioner will need to decrease the angle of the needle to prevent puncturing of the posterior wall of the vein. The cannula can then be advanced a few millimetres into the vein to ensure that the tip of the needle and the tip of the cannula trim are sitting in the vein lumen.

Traction must be maintained on the vein with the non-dominant hand while the practitioner gently withdraws the needle back into the trim of the cannula (approximately 3 mm). The practitioner will encounter a second 'flashback' of blood; this is the blood from the vein flowing up the cannula shaft which indicates that the cannula can now be advanced fully into the vein. The non-dominant hand then anchors the skin, securing the stylet with the thumb and index finger. If at this stage the second flashback is not observed, the stylet should not be reintroduced as this could result in the cannula tip being sheared off by the stylet with the potential of causing a catheter embolism (Perucca 2010). Once the cannula has been fully advanced into the vein, the tourniquet can be released. Pressure is then applied with the non-dominant hand above the cannula using the index finger to anchor the cannula with the middle and fourth finger occluding the blood flow immediately above the cannula. Only when the stylet has been safely removed, resulting in a third flash of blood in the final collection chamber before connection of injection cap or extension set, can the practitioner be assured of achieving a successful cannulation.

If the one-handed method is used, the hand that performs the cannulation also withdraws the stylet and advances the cannula into the vein, whilst maintaining skin traction with the non-dominant hand. This can be more difficult for the practitioner to learn but once this method has been acquired can result in a better success rate (Dougherty 2008). The two-handed technique is when the practitioner uses the dominant hand to perform the cannulation and the middle and ring fingers of the non-dominant hand to maintain the skin traction; once the practitioner has identified blood in the cannula chamber they use the thumb and index finger of the non-dominant hand to grip the stylet, and keeping the traction constant the stylet is then withdrawn slightly using the non dominant thumb and index finger, and the dominant hand advances the cannula off the stylet.

Equipment required to perform cannulation

- Clinically clean tray or receiver
- Disposable tourniquet
- 2% Chlorhexidine with 70% alcohol impregnated swabs
- Appropriate dressing and securement device
- Cannula of various gauge sizes
- 0.9% sodium chloride solution for flushing

- Sterile cotton wool or gauze
- Tape or adhesive plaster
- Sterile dressing pack

- 5 mL syringe

- Clinically clean gloves

- Sharps bin

Cannulation procedure

The practitioner will need to consider what type of therapy is being infused as this will influence the type and gauge of cannula to be used, as well as the location the cannula is to be sited. They will also need to establish the anticipated duration of the prescribed therapy. On no account should the practitioner attempt to amend an unsuccessful cannulation by reinserting the stylet needle (Perucca 2010). If the practitioner has more than two attempts, unnecessary trauma is caused to the patient and resultant multiple puncture sites may render the vein unusable for cannulation at a later time (Phillips 2005). Always consider if a cannula is really necessary; sometimes a cannula can be inserted routinely 'just in case' and this practice should be challenged (Wait *et al.* 2004).

Step	Action	Rationale
Preparation		
1	Prepare the area by considering, the lighting, privacy, local temperature and equipment to be used.	To ensure that the patient as well as the practitioner are adequately prepared.
2	Position patient on a chair or couch.	To maintain safety of patient if they experience vasovagal faint. Also for patient's comfort.
3	Ensure patient's correct identity by asking patient to state their name or check identification bracelet.	To ensure procedure is being performed on the correct patient (NPSA 2006).

4	Give thorough explanation of the procedure, allowing time for the patient to address any questions and discuss any previous difficulties that may have arisen. Consult cannula care plan if documentation available.	To obtain consent and in discussing patient's previous history consider the most appropriate equipment to perform the procedure effectively (Lavery 2003).
5	Apply topical local anaesthetic if required.	To give adequate time for topical local anaesthetic to take effect (BMA & RPS 2011).
6	Ask the patient which arm they would prefer and position patient's arm by supporting on a pillow.	To maintain comfort.
7	Collect sufficient quantities of all necessary equipment (see list above).	To avoid any unnecessary interruptions during the procedure.
8	Ensure that packaging has been checked with seals intact, and that none of the equipment has passed the expiry date.	To avoid the risk of using faulty or contaminated equipment.

9	Perform effective hand washing technique using soap and water or appropriate alcohol rub.	To minimise the risk of infection and maintain asepsis (Franklin 1999; Hindley 2004).
10	Cover any visibly broken skin on the practitioner with a suitable waterproof dressing.	To reduce the risk of contamination by blood to the practitioner.
11	Take tray or trolley containing all necessary equipment selected to perform the procedure to patient's bedside.	To avoid any unnecessary interruptions during the procedure.

Vein assessment and selection

| 12 | Apply tourniquet 7–8 cm above desired location. | To create adequate venous filling (RCN 2010). |
| 13 | To assist venous filling, the patient can:

(a) Clench fist.
(b) Lower the arm downwards, over side of couch or bed.
(c) Finally to assist venous filling the patient can immerse the limb into a bowl of hot water. | To aid venous filling and increase the prominence of patient's veins in order to ascertain the direction of the vein's pathway and its depth and identify any surrounding structures that need to be avoided tendons and arteries. |

14	Assess the patient's veins examining and palpating them whilst selecting appropriate site.	To avoid discomfort to patient and prevent unsuccessful cannulation.
15	Release the tourniquet.	To maintain patient's comfort
16	If the chosen site is covered/obscured by hair growth the practitioner may consider removing this with scissors or clippers.	To reduce risk of infection (Weinstein 2007) and facilitate the adherence of the dressing.
17	Wash hands with bacterial soap and water or bacterial alcohol handrub.	To minimise the risk of infection (DH 2005).
18	Open sterile pack and assemble equipment, selecting the appropriate gauge and length of cannula and prime the needle-free extension set if required.	To be equipped with the most suitable gauge of cannula to perform the procedure effectively and reduce any unnecessary trauma to the veins (Lavery 2003).
19	Reapply tourniquet.	To create adequate venous filling and to increase prominence of veins by obstructing venous return.

20	Clean the skin for minimum of 30 seconds with a 2% chlorhexidine-based solution. Ensure that the cleaning action is directed over the entire site which will be covered by the cannula dressing and has been delivered using sufficient pressure to remove surface dirt and debris. The skin should then be allowed to air dry for minimum of 30 seconds. The skin should not be re-palpated or the site touched once this has taken place.	To maintain asepsis (DH 2007).
21	Put on gloves.	To minimise risk of infection by forming a protective layer against any blood spillage (ICNA 2003).
22	Remove needle guard. Inspect the cannula to determine that there are no faults.	To ensure equipment is intact and free of faults (MHRA 2005; RCN 2010).
23	Hold the device, depending on type of cannula and technique to be adopted.	

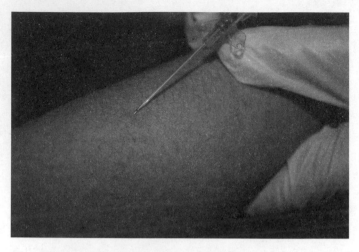

Fig. 7.11 Bevel of needle uppermost to smooth entry into skin and vein (skin entry view).

24	Ensure that the bevel of the needle is in correct position, i.e. uppermost (Fig. 7.11).	To facilitate smooth entry into vein and reduce trauma to skin and vein on entry. To ensure correct positioning between needle point and cannula trim.

Insertion

25	Anchor the vein by applying traction a few centimetres below the proposed insertion site ensuring that the skin is not touched. This traction needs to be maintained throughout the procedure (Fig. 7.12 and Fig. 7.13).	To anchor vein in order to immobilise and provide counter tension to facilitate smoother needle entry. Ensure anchoring is not released too early, as this could result in the needle penetrating the opposing vein wall.

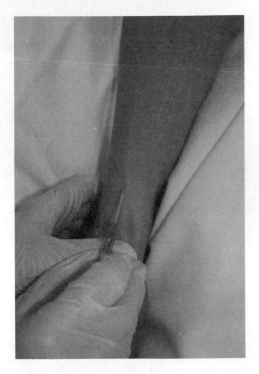

Fig. 7.12 Anchor vein throughout procedure.

26   According to the depth of the vein the needle should be inserted at the practitioner's discretion between an angle of 10 and 40 degrees (Figs 7.13).

To indicate that the needle has penetrated the vein. To reduce risk of penetration of the distal wall of the vein with the cannula needle.

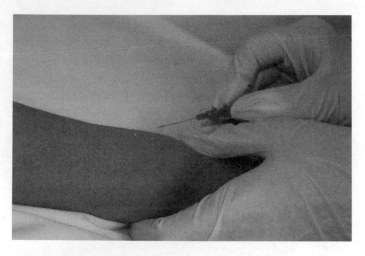

Fig. 7.13 Angle of insertion of cannula.

27   Once flashback is seen in the flashback chamber (Fig. 7.14a and b), lower the angle of the cannula and advance the cannula a few millimetres into the vein.

To ensure that the distance between the bevel of the needle and the trim has entered the lumen of the vein.

28   Withdraw stylet 1–2 mm and identify a second flashback of blood as it feeds back along the cannula (Fig. 7.15).

To ensure that cannula is in situ so can be safely advanced into lumen of vein.

(a)

(b)

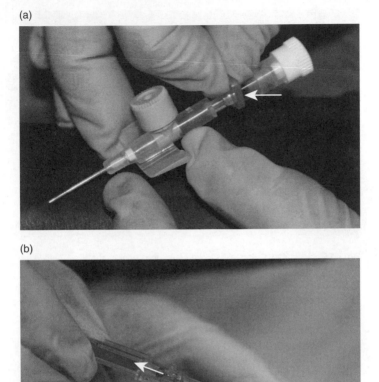

Fig. 7.14 (a) Primary flashback (see arrow) – blood enters the cannula. Used with permission of Vein Train Ltd. (b) Primary flashback (see arrow) – first flashback into needle and flashback chamber of a nonported cannula.

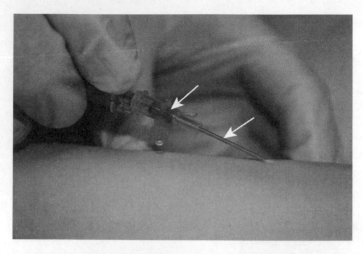

Fig. 7.15 Secondary flashback – blood enters the cannula shaft (see arrows).

29	Firmly hold the stylet to avoid accidental reinsertion of stylet.	To immobilise the needle and prevent stylet being reinserted, which may result in the needle damaging the cannula with potential risk of causing a catheter embolus.
30	Slowly advance the cannula ensuring that the vein remains anchored during the procedure. (Fig. 7.16)	To detect any resistance that may be experienced, e.g. valves.
31	Release the tourniquet.	To decrease the pressure within the vein.

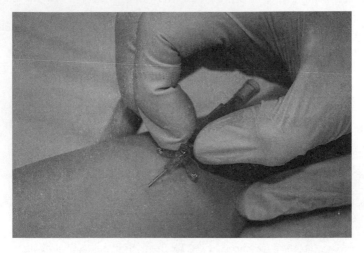

Fig. 7.16 Advance cannula into vein.

Completion and disposal

32	Apply digital pressure to the vein above the cannula, ensuring that the cannula is also anchored.	To prevent spillage of blood.
33	Remove the stylet and discard immediately into sharps bin.	To prevent needlestick injury to practitioner or patient.
34	Connect the needle-free injection cap or primed extension set to end of cannula.	To prevent entry of bacteria and prevent blood spillage.

35	Flush cannula with 5 ml of 0.9% sodium chloride (prescribed or under patient group direction). It should be flushed according to local policy using a push–pause technique and ending with positive pressure to prevent backflow of blood into the cannula (Dougherty 2008).	To maintain patency.
36	Observe for signs of swelling or leakage and ask the patient if they are experiencing any pain or discomfort.	To check that the cannula is in the vein (RCN 2010).
37	Secure the cannula with an appropriate securement device and an appropriate dressing.	To secure cannula thus preventing movement and reducing the risk of irritation of the vein wall, which could result in the development of mechanical phlebitis. To allow ongoing inspection of the cannula site and prevent entry of microorganisms between cannula and skin.
38	Remove gloves.	To prevent cross-contamination.

| 39 | Dispose of clinical waste in the appropriate container. | To ensure staff safety and comply with universal precautions. |
| 40 | Document the insertion procedure in care pathway, care plan or nursing notes. Ensure that the date, time, gauge and location of cannula are all recorded together with the number of attempts and the signature of the practitioner who inserted the device. | To maintain professional accountability. To establish how long the cannula has been sited, and to help to identify where they have been previously sited (DH 2007). |

Troubleshooting

A number of problems can occur during cannulation. The practitioner should consider the following potential reasons for unsuccessful insertion.

No initial flashback

Cause	Prevention	Action
Needle may not have penetrated far enough into the vein through the subcutaneous tissue.	Angle of entry may not have been steep enough. Review the angle of approach.	Slowly advance the needle and observe for a flashback, observe how much of the needle has been inserted into the vein.

Cannula may have made contact with a valve.	Difficult to identify location of valve on palpation. Avoid areas in dorsal vein where two veins bifurcate.	Withdraw the cannula slightly to distance it from valve.
Vein too small.	Avoid where possible, reassess or relocate to a different site.	Consider the use of the indirect method of cannulation.
Slow flashback of blood in the cannula chamber when using a smaller gauge cannula.		Allow up to 20 seconds for the flashback to appear in the chamber of the cannula.

No second flashback

Cause	Prevention
Trim of cannula not fully inserted into the vein.	Ensure needle is advanced 1–2 mm after initial flashback (to ensure cannula also in vein) before attempting to glide cannula off the needle.
Needle and cannula transfixed through the other side of the vein	Decrease angle of cannula to prevent puncturing the posterior wall of the vein.

If on entry blood is observed to leak around the needle
The practitioner should consider:

Cause	Prevention	Action
Practitioner advancing cannula stylet too slowly and bevel of needle contacts vein before fully under skin.	Improve technique.	Adopt a confident swift approach into proposed cannulation site. Tourniquet may be too tight.

CARE AND MANAGEMENT OF CANNULA IN SITU
The cannulated patient is well placed to be the first person to recognise any symptoms that might indicate a problem affecting the management of the cannula placement. Providing patients with an information leaflet to read before they have their cannula inserted is a useful tool, and this knowledge will empower the patient. It should contain a full explanation of the cannula, why or what it is used for, and describe symptoms that may be experienced should the cannula become problematic.

Once a cannula has been successfully sited it is important that it is adequately secured with tape or a securing device e.g. Statlock to prevent mechanical phlebitis or accidental dislodgement. If the cannula has been secured using clean tape, care needs to be taken that it does not come in contact with the insertion site. Cannulae can be covered with dry sterile gauze and transparent dressings to secure and protect the device (Dougherty 2008). Covering cannula sites with bandages should be avoided, as they inhibit observation of the site making it difficult to identify problems. Where patients are very young or to promote patient safety it may become necessary to secure the cannula to maintain skin integrity (Finlay 2008). A small splint can also be used when a cannula has been inserted near a flexion point (Finlay 2004).

Once inserted a primed needle-free extension set can be attached. Most of these systems allow the attachment of intermittent infusions, without removing the cap and thereby maintaining a closed system minimising risk of infection (Weinstein

2007). Care needs to be taken to clean the needle-free connector, and to allow it to air dry for 30 seconds every time the system is accessed. Once sited the cannula should be flushed with sodium chloride 0.9%. This should be continued prior to and after each use. If a cannula is being left in situ, it requires flushing every 24 hours to maintain patency (Campbell *et al.* 2005).

An accurate record of care must be documented at regular intervals throughout the duration of the cannula placement. The practitioner should document the insertion according to local policy. Documentation must include the date (DH 2003), time (RCN 2010) and any problems encountered during insertion. It should also include device size (Dougherty 2008), the insertion site including actual vein(s) used (Dougherty 2008; Pellowe *et al.* 2007; Weinstein 2007) and the name of the person placing the device (RCN 2010). Recording of batch numbers is also recommended (INS 2006). The practitioner needs to observe the insertion site, and maintain an ongoing record of the cannula site. This information needs to be documented on every shift. Ensure any infusion sets connected to the cannula are also labelled with the date when they were first attached. A useful tool to support documentation of the cannula site is the visual infusion phlebitis scoring system or cannula care plan (see Chapter 8).

Educating all members of the multidisciplinary team to recognise problems affecting cannula management is essential. Cannulae can be left in situ safely between 72 and 96 hours, providing vigilant assessment and documentation is maintained (DH 2007).

PROCEDURE FOR SAFE REMOVAL OF CANNULA

Prior to removing a cannula the patient has to be prepared and an explanation of the procedure given to reassure them.

The practitioner will need to gather together the following equipment:

- clinically clean tray or receiver
- clinically clean gloves
- sterile gauze and tape.

	Action	**Rationale**
1	Perform effective hand washing technique or using soap and water appropriate alcohol rub.	To minimise the risk of infection and maintain asepsis (Franklin 1999; Hindley 2004)
2	Put on clinically clean gloves.	To minimise risk of infection by forming a protective layer against any blood spillage (ICNA 2003).
3	Carefully remove dressing.	To avoid any trauma to the insertion site of cannula.
4	Open sterile gauze.	To ensure practitioner is adequately prepared.
5	Gently withdraw cannula from the site; pressure should not be applied until the cannula has been fully removed.	To avoid causing pain to the patient and to facilitate easy exit of cannula, avoiding trauma to cannula site.
6	Apply digital pressure to the site for 1–2 minutes with the sterile gauze.	To prevent leakage, preserve vein and avoid haematoma.
7	Inspect the cannula site and if bleeding has discontinued cover with an appropriate dressing.	To ensure there is no further bleeding. To check that the puncture site is covered with a suitable dressing after checking the patients allergy status.

8	Inspect cannula.	To ensure that it has been fully removed and check for length and integrity (RCN 2010).
9	Dispose of cannula and dressing.	To prevent cross contamination.
10	Document the date, time and reason for removal of the cannula.	To maintain professional accountability and establish how long the cannula has been in situ (DH 2007; RCN 2010).

CONCLUSION

Safe preparation of the environment, practitioner and patient will enable venepuncture and cannulation to be performed efficiently and safely with minimal discomfort to the patient. With consistent supervision at the outset the practitioner will achieve the dexterity and confidence required to perform these skills successfully. When embarking on the challenge posed by patients with depleted venous access, experience gained by awareness of appropriate troubleshooting techniques will increase the proficiency of the practitioner.

REFERENCES

Black, F. & Hughes, J. (1997) Venepuncture. *Nursing Standard*, **11**(41), 49–53.

BMA & RPS (2011) *British National Formulary*. British Medical Association and Royal Pharmaceutical Society, London.

Campbell, S.G., Trojanowski, J. & Ackroyd-Stolarz, S.A. (2005) How often should intravenous catheters in ambulatory patients be flushed? *Journal of Infusion Nursing*, **28**(6), 399–404.

Davies, J. & Aston, D. (2002) Inappropriate blood transfusions caused by poor phlebotomy techniques. *Transfusion Medicine*, **12**(Supplement 11), 38.

Department of Health (2003) *Winning Ways. Working Together to Reduce Healthcare Associated Infection in England*. Department of Health Publications

Department of Health (DH) (2005) *Hazardous Waste (England) Regulations*. DH, London.

Department of Health (DH) (2007) *Saving Lives: High Impact Intervention No 2, Peripheral intravenous cannula care bundle*. DH, London.

Dougherty, L. (2008) Obtaining peripheral venous access. In: *Intravenous Therapy in Nursing Practice* (eds L. Dougherty & J. Lamb), 2nd edn, pp. 225–270. Blackwell Publishing, Oxford.

Finlay, T. (2004) *Intravenous Therapy*. Blackwell Publishing. Oxford.

Finlay, T. (2008) Safe administration and management of peripheral intravenous therapy. In: *Intravenous Therapy in Nursing Practice* (eds L. Dougherty & J. Lamb), 2nd edn, pp. 143–166. Blackwell Publishing, Oxford.

Franklin, L. (1999) Skin cleansing and infection control in peripheral venepuncture and cannulation. *Nursing Standard*, **14**(4), 49–50.

Health Protection Agency (2005) *Eye of the Needle*. HPA. England.

Hindley, G. (2004) Handwashing Infection control in peripheral cannula. *Nursing Standard*, **18**(37), 37–40.

Infection Control Nurses Association (ICNA) (2003) *Reducing sharps injury – prevention and risk management*. Infection Control Nurse Association, February.

INS (2006) Infusion Nursing Standards of Practice. *Journal of Infusion Nursing*, **29**(1 Supp) S1–S92.

Lavery, I. (2003) Peripheral intravenous cannulation and patient consent. *Nursing Standard*, **17**(28), 40-42.

Lavery, I. & Ingram, P. (2005) Venepuncture: best practice. *Nursing Standard*, **19**(49), 55–65.

McCall, R.E. & Tankersley, C.M. (2008) *Phlebotomy Essentials*, 4th edn. Lippincott Williams & Wilkins, Philadelphia.

MDA – Medicines and Healthcare Products Regulatory Agency (2001) *Safe use and disposal of sharps*. MDA SN, 2001(19).

MHRA (2005) *Alert MDA 2005/01 and Device bulletin DB 2005 (01). Reporting adverse incidents and disseminating medical device alerts*. Medicines and Healthcare Products Agency, London.

National Patient Safety Agency (NPSA) (2006). *Right patient right blood. Safer Practice Notice 14*. NPSA, London.

NBS (2007) *Requirements for Sample Labelling and Request Form Completion*. NBS Policy MPD/DDR/DD/009/03, 2007.

NBS – National Blood Service (2008) *Transfusion Matters: The Journey of a Bag of Blood from Hospital Laboratory to Patient*, 5th edn (Summer/Autumn), pp. 1–4.

Pellowe, C.M., Pratt, R.J., Loveday, H.P., Harper, P., Robinson, N. & Jones, S.R.L.J. (2007) The epic project. Updating the evidence base for national evidence-based guidelines for preventing healthcare associated infections in NHS hospitals in England: a report with recommendations. *Journal of Infection Control*, **5**(6), 10–16.

Perucca R. (2010) Peripheral venous access devices. In: *Infusion Nursing: An evidence based approach* (eds M. Alexander, A. Corrigan, L. Gorski, J. Hankins & R. Perucca), 3rd edn. pp. 456–479. Saunders Elsevier, Philadelphia.

Phillips, L. (2005) *Manual of IV Therapeutics*, 4th edn. FA Davis, Philadelphia.

RCN (2010) *Standard for Infusion Therapy*, 3rd edn. RCN, London.

Springhouse (2002) *Intravenous Therapy Made Incredibly Easy*, 2nd edn. Lippincott Williams & Wilkins, Philadelphia.

Wait, G., Waitt, P. & Pirmohamed, M. (2004) Intravenous therapy. *Postgraduate Medical Journal*, **80**(939), 1–6.

Weinstein, S.M. (2007) *Plumer's Principles and Practice of Infusion Therapy*, 8th edn. Lippincott Williams & Wilkins, Philadelphia.

Complications

8

Wendy Morris

LEARNING OUTCOMES

The practitioner will be able to:
- ❏ List the most common complications of venepuncture and cannulation.
- ❏ Identify the predisposing factors for these complications.
- ❏ Explain the management for each of these complications.

INTRODUCTION

Venepuncture and cannulation are commonly performed procedures within healthcare practice, and in the majority of instances used without complication to treat patients. However, each time these procedures are performed there is potential for the patient to experience trauma to their veins. Problems range from slight bruising to economic impact as a result of infection and in extreme cases death. Complications may arise at different stages of the procedure: on initial assessment when attempting to source a suitable site to insert the vascular device, or subsequently during the insertion procedure, or later during care of the site/device.

The potential for development of complications at these stages may be influenced by a number of contributory factors: the ageing process, gender, vein selection, equipment selection, disease processes, treatment protocols and the skill of the

Venepuncture and Cannulation, first edition. Edited by Sarah Phillips,
Mary Collins and Lisa Dougherty. Published 2011 by Blackwell Publishing Ltd.
© 2011 Blackwell Publishing Ltd.

practitioner. In order to prevent these problems occurring, healthcare providers implement strategies to prevent complications occurring, reduce patient morbidity, and improve skills of healthcare professionals (Collins *et al.* 2006; Morris & Tay 2008). It is therefore important that practitioners are equipped with sound vascular knowledge to anticipate potential complications and possess the ability to competently and professionally manage each complication as it arises. It is also important that the patient's consent for the procedure is obtained prior to undertaking either procedure (DH 2001a, b).

Within this chapter the most common complications of venepuncture and cannulation will be discussed. Strategies to prevent and manage these occurrences will also be provided.

ECCHYMOSIS/HAEMATOMA

Ecchymosis is a term to describe the infiltration of blood into tissue (Perucca 2010). Haematoma describes bleeding (usually uncontrolled) which occurs as a result of infiltration of blood from a punctured vein into the tissue immediately surrounding it, resulting in a painful swelling; this is the most common complication of venepuncture (McCall & Tankersley 2008). Ecchymosis occurs first, then if bleeding continues a haematoma will form. A haematoma can be recognised as a purple/blue-tinged lump at the point of needle insertion, which starts off small and becomes larger. Once a haematoma has formed it cannot be rectified; the procedure should be aborted and the haematoma managed.

Specific predisposing factors for haematoma formation

- Poor practitioner technique: a tentative stop–start technique which injures the vein, often associated with beginners (Weinstein 2007).
- Vulnerable patient groups such as: the young/elderly and those on anticoagulant therapy (RCN 2010).
- Poor vein selection: use of fine or thready veins, sites too near valves, or using a needle too large for the chosen vein (McCall & Tankersley 2008; Dimech *et al.* 2011).

- Failure to release the tourniquet before removing the device (Lavery & Ingram 2005); as a result high intravascular pressure causes bleeding outside the vein.
- Failure to insert the needle correctly into the vein, or poor device manipulation following puncture of a vein, causing the needle to pierce the distal vein wall (Campbell *et al.* 1999).
- Application of a tourniquet to a limb in order to undertake a second attempt to insert a vascular device, within a short period of time of the initial attempt (Weinstein 2007).
- Multiple attempts to access a vein, or when attempting to access veins that are difficult to visualise or palpate (Perucca 2010).

Prevention of haematoma

Preventative action	Rationale
Avoid performing venepuncture/cannulation at a haematoma site.	To prevent causing the patient pain and delaying healing at the puncture site. Venepuncture samples taken from a haematoma site may produce inaccurate blood results due to contamination from haemolysed blood within the bruise (McCall & Tankersley 2008).
Be aware of the patient's medical history. Any predisposing factors which may cause bleeding for extended periods e.g. anticoagulant/ steroid therapy.	To anticipate complications and identify the most appropriate equipment for the procedure.

Preventative action

Be aware of patient groups who are at risk of haematoma formation. For instance the ageing process results in a reduction of subcutaneous tissue and a reduction in skin elasticity which makes veins and skin more friable.

Rationale

To anticipate at-risk patient groups

Use the smallest sized device suitable for the procedure, and try to avoid small fragile veins. Consider the needs of the patient, number of samples required (venepuncture) location of the device and the infusion solution to be administered (cannulation) (Dougherty 2008a).

To reduce the potential for haematoma formation.

Place all equipment within easy reach.

To prevent unnecessary stretching by the practitioner which may cause the hand (holding the vascular device) to move and force the needle through the vein wall or, accidentally pull the needle out of the vein.

Using the non-dominant hand anchor the vein securely below the proposed puncture site. Ensure the bevel of the venepuncture needle/ cannula is upright and introduce the vascular device smoothly through the skin, while continuing to maintain firm skin traction.

Firm skin traction prevents the skin puckering, the vein rolling (missed vein entry), and is less painful for the patient (Dougherty 2008a).

Preventative action	**Rationale**
Once the vein has been successfully accessed, keep the needle static. Rest fingers lightly on the patient's limb to prevent movement when inserting and removing blood bottles (venepuncture).	Movement of a needle whilst in a vein increases the potential for piercing the distal vein wall causing haematoma formation.
Apply firm skin traction at the base of the vein chosen to insert the cannula into. Maintain firm skin traction throughout the procedure until the cannula has been successfully inserted into the vein.	To immobilise the vein, ensuring the cannula stylet does not pierce the distal vein wall when the cannula is being threaded off the stylet into the vein.
Following removal of a vascular device care for the puncture site according to local policy. Apply firm pressure with a sterile dressing to the puncture site until bleeding has ceased and haemostasis is achieved (Dougherty 2008a; Dimech *et al.* 2011).	Insufficient pressure applied to a puncture site allows bleeding to continue beneath the skin, which may result in haematoma formation, with the potential for nerve injury and reflex sympathetic dystrophy to develop (Weinstein 2007).
If the first attempt to gain venous access is unsuccessful, consider using the opposite limb for the subsequent attempt (according to local policy).	Application of a tourniquet increases venous pressure. This may cause a recently punctured vein, e.g. due to an unsuccessful venous access attempt or recently removed vascular device, to start rebleeding, increasing the potential for haematoma formation (Weinstein 2007).

Preventative action

Rationale

Before leaving the patient inspect the puncture site to ensure bleeding has ceased.

To ensure the puncture site has been correctly cared for.

If the patient has fragile skin, e.g. if the patient is elderly, consider applying the tourniquet over a layer of clothing or a clinical dressing.

To reduce the potential for the tourniquet to cause skin abrasions resulting in ecchymosis/bruising of the skin.

Alternatively, ask a colleague to act as a tourniquet by wrapping their hands around the limb and squeezing gently.

To encourage venous dilation while reducing the potential for ecchymosis/haematoma.

If a new cannula has to be inserted into a limb in which an existing cannula is currently in situ (because it has not been previously removed), insert the new cannula above the old, then remove the unnecessary cannula.

Application of a tourniquet to a limb which has had a vascular device recently removed may cause the puncture site to start rebleeding.

Site new cannula above valves.

The presence of valves may prevent a cannula being advanced through a vein. Application of force to push the cannula through the valve may cause pain, or result in the needle piercing and rupturing the distal vein wall, causing haematoma formation.

Management of haematoma

Action	Rationale
Observe for a blue/purple lump at the puncture site when inserting the vascular device.	To identify haematoma formation.
On recognition of a haematoma immediately release the tourniquet, cease the procedure and remove the vascular device according to local policy.	A tourniquet generates and maintains high venous pressure, making it easier to palpate veins prior to gaining venous access (Dimech *et al.* 2011). Failure to release the tourniquet after recognition of a haematoma causes bleeding to persist into tissue surrounding the puncture site.
Remove the vascular device, using a sterile swab, apply digital pressure to puncture site until bleeding has ceased and haemostasis is achieved (Dougherty 2008a).	To stem bleeding from the puncture site on removal of device. Application of digital pressure at the puncture site prior to removing the needle can cause the needle tip to drag against the tunica intima, damaging the lining of the vein and causing acute pain (Dimech *et al.* 2011). If the patient is receiving anticoagulant therapy, or suffering disease processes which interfere with their clotting mechanisms, pressure may need to be applied to the puncture site for an extended period.

Action	**Rationale**
Following puncture of a vein at the antecubital fossa or removal of a cannula from this site advise the patient not to bend their arm upwards towards their face whilst simultaneously applying pressure to the puncture site (Ernst 2005).	Bending the arm upwards interferes with application of digital pressure to the site, allowing blood to leak into surrounding tissue.
If bleeding persists elevate the affected limb. If necessary apply ice to the puncture site.	Application of ice promotes vasoconstriction and cessation of bleeding.
Provide the patient with an information leaflet explaining what has occurred; discuss any concerns.	To inform and reassure the patient.
Instruct the patient to contact a doctor if they become concerned about the haematoma site, e.g. increasing pain, enlarging haematoma.	Pain may be indicative that blood from the haematoma site has accumulated and is pressing on a nerve (McCall & Tankersley 2008).
Document the incident in the clinical notes.	To provide evidence of haematoma formation and actions taken to treat the site.
If appropriate apply Hirudoid cream or arnica cream (as per manufacturer's instructions) to the haematoma site.	To encourage healing.

Action	Rationale
Before leaving the patient inspect the puncture site to ensure bleeding has ceased.	To provide care of the site.
After removing the venepuncture needle/ cannula and achieving haemostasis do not interfere with the puncture site again.	To prevent the therapeutic clot sealing the puncture site being disturbed, resulting in rebleeding at the site.
Prior to venous access, assess the equipment and technique necessary to undertake the procedure. Consider if an alternative venous access device could be used, e.g. butterfly for venepuncture rather than vacutainer needle, or if a central venous access device (CVAD) should be inserted for long-term vascular therapy.	Becoming a skilled practitioner involves reflecting upon past procedures and recognising how they can be improved upon.

MISSED VEIN

Insufficient traction of the vein during insertion of the vascular device can result in missing the vein. Insufficient traction allows the vein to roll (move away) when the needle is inserted, causing it to lie parallel with the vein rather than piercing it. This may be a particular problem with some patient groups, such as elderly people who as part of the ageing process experience a loss of subcutaneous tissue which would normally serve to stabilise veins. The practitioner may find that when skin traction is applied the vein moves beneath the skin, making it difficult to identify where the vascular device should be inserted. In this instance the vascular device insertion point will need to be adjusted to accommodate movement of the vein. Practitioners have been known to inform patients that 'their veins move', causing some to believe they have a vascular problem. In reality, missing a vein is usually due to poor practitioner technique and difficulty stabilizing a vein.

Specific predisposing factors for missing a vein

- Poor skin stabilisation (Dougherty 2008a).
- Poor vein choice or failure to penetrate the vein due to a poor insertion angle (McCall & Tankersley 2008).
- The ageing process; which decreases the amount of subcutaneous tissue available to support a vein (Weinstein 2007).

Prevention of 'missing a vein'

Preventative action	Rationale
Choose the most suitable vascular access device. Use the smallest device appropriate for the procedure.	To increase the potential for one successful attempt and limit damage to the vein.
Apply tourniquet and palpate the chosen vein to assess its suitability. The most prominent vein is not always the most suitable.	To increase the potential of a successful procedure.
Prior to inserting the vascular device apply and remove skin traction a few times beneath the chosen puncture site.	To enable the practitioner to identify whether the vein moves position when traction is applied. This enables the practitioner to adjust the proposed insertion site to accommodate movement of the vein.

Preventative action	**Rationale**
Using the non-dominant hand anchor the vein securely below the proposed puncture site. Ensure the bevel of the venepuncture needle/cannula is upright, aim for the middle of vein and introduce the vascular device smoothly through the skin into the vein.	Firm skin traction immobilises the vein preventing the skin puckering and the vein rolling (missed vein entry), and is less painful for the patient when the vascular device is inserted (Dougherty 2008a).
Maintain firm skin traction throughout the procedure.	Stabilising the vein sufficiently is extremely important and will influence success or failure. If the vein is not well supported the tip of the vascular device may be unable to pierce the vein, instead nudging it out of position and causing the needle tip to sit in subcutaneous tissue and lie parallel with the vein rather than piercing it.
Look for blood flowing into blood collection bottle (venepuncture) or flashback in the chamber (cannulation), then complete the procedure.	Evidence the vein has been successfully punctured.
If using veins on the back of the hand. Ask the patient to make a fist, then extend it down towards the floor.	To assist with immobilising dorsal veins, making them less likely to roll away from the vascular device when it is inserted.

Preventative action

If the patient has small fine veins employ techniques, e.g. application of heat, to encourage venous dilation and use the smallest sized needle/cannula for the procedure.

Rationale

To encourage venous dilation and the potential for one successful attempt at venous access.

Management if a vein is missed

Action

No blood flow into blood bottles (venepuncture), no flashback in chamber (cannulation).

Rationale

Problem identified.

Remove blood collection bottles from vacutainer holder (venepuncture).

To maintain blood bottle vacuum, so that the blood collection bottles can be reused on the same patient.

Keep the dominant hand immobile to prevent the vacutainer needle/ cannula moving within the tissue.

To prevent the practitioner accidentally pulling the vascular device out of the vein or causing the patient pain.

Using your palpation finger, palpate the vein above the puncture site. Feel where the needle lies in relation to the vein.

To establish if the procedure can be rectified.

Provide traction at the base of the vein to immobilise it. This will prevent the vein rolling further away from the needle when the vascular device is manipulated.

To increase the potential of completing the procedure.

Action	**Rationale**
Pull the vascular device slightly out of the skin (take care not to pull it out completely). Reapply firm skin traction to the base of the vein. Carefully realign the needle tip and if able, reinsert the vascular device into the skin at an angle capable of piercing the side of the vein wall.	To attempt to rectify the procedure.
Observe for blood draining into the blood collection bottle (venepuncture) or visible in the flashback chamber (cannulation), then complete the procedure.	Evidence the procedure has been successful.
If at any point in the procedure the patient complains of pain, abort the procedure.	To prevent causing undue discomfort or nerve damage.
Never introduce the needle blindly into areas where you think the vein may be.	To prevent the needle being pushed further into soft tissue, blind probing increases the potential for haematoma formation, nerve damage and pain.
If the vein moves a large distance it may be necessary to provide traction at the base of the vein pulling downwards (vertically) whilst simultaneously stretching the skin horizontally using thumb and forefinger.	To provide skin traction in two directions in order to immobilise the vein.

VASOVAGAL/SYNCOPE REACTION

For some individuals undergoing intravenous therapy fear of pain, needles and confinement generates anxiety. In extreme instances this may result in individuals failing to access healthcare facilities, resulting in serious repercussions. For others this fear may manifest itself as vasovagal syncope or loss of consciousness in the presence of needles (Deacon & Abramowitz 2006). This reaction may be influenced by poor previous experiences, or the attitudes of healthcare professionals, both of which influence an individual's perception of the procedure (Weinstein 2007). Exaggerated fears have the potential to create a negative autonomic nervous system response known as a vasovagal response, which may manifest itself as syncope. Although usually benign and self-limiting there is potential for the sufferer to experience injury if an episode is not anticipated. An episode may prove embarrassing for the patient and stressful for the healthcare professional caring for the patient. Symptoms commonly experienced include light-headedness, fainting, nausea, feeling hot or cold or sweaty. A sympathetic response may develop causing vasoconstriction and collapse of veins, depleting the number of veins available for vascular access and causing the procedure to become more complicated (Weinstein 2007).

Specific predisposing factors to vasovagal/syncope reaction

- Fear of needles or blood (Weinstein 2007).
- Family history of needle phobia or vasovagal reactions (Ost 1991).
- Learnt response; parents conveying fear to their children (Willemsen *et al.* 2002).
- Feeling unwell (Weinstein 2007).
- Poor previous experiences (Lavery & Ingram 2005).

Prevention of vasovagal/syncope reaction

Preventative action	Rationale
The practitioner must behave in a calm confident manner.	To instil confidence in the patient about the skill of the practitioner.
Provide the patient with concise information about the procedure and respond to questions clearly.	To reduce anxiety.
While preparing the patient for the procedure, establish if they have ever experienced problems when in close proximity with needles or possess a fear of needles or blood.	To anticipate problems prior to their occurrence and implement safety precautions.
If the patient is anxious and the practitioner inexperienced, consider asking an experienced colleague to perform the procedure.	Anxious patients can make inexperienced practitioners feel nervous; making it less likely the procedure will be successful.
Only experienced practitioners should attempt venepuncture/cannulation on anxious patients, especially if they have difficult venous access (Weinstein 2007).	Experienced practitioners are more successful at performing vascular procedures (Weinstein 2007).
If the patient experiences anxiety around needles/blood lay them flat.	To ensure patient safety.
Ask the patient how they normally manage their reaction to needles and blood. Encourage the patient to practise deep breathing exercises. Suggest the individual looks in the opposite direction when performing the procedure.	To employ coping mechanisms.

Preventative action	Rationale
Involve the patient in finding a suitable vein.	To encourage the individual to feel in control of the procedure and reduce anxiety.
Consider the use of topical anaesthetic, e.g. EMLA/Ametop cream prior to inserting the vascular device (Lavery & Ingram 2005).	To lessen the pain and anxiety associated with the procedure (Scales, 2005).
When using topical anaesthetic take time to find the most appropriate vein prior to applying the anaesthetic cream/gel. Veins that are palpable are often more suitable than veins that can be easily observed.	To locate the most appropriate site to insert the vascular device.
If appropriate allow the patient to have a family/friend accompany them during the procedure. First check family members/friends themselves do not possess a needle/blood phobia.	Anxious/needle-phobic friends/relatives will increase anxiety levels experienced by the patient undergoing the procedure, making the procedure more difficult to perform.
Talk to the individual in a calm manner throughout the procedure until it is completed.	To reduce anxiety and distract the patient during the procedure, thereby reducing the potential for a sympathetic nervous response to occur causing veins to constrict making the procedure more difficult (flight or fight response).

Management of syncope/vasovagal reaction

Action	Rationale
Anticipate if the patient may faint. If practical lay the person flat on a couch/ bed prior to commencing the procedure.	To ensure patient safety.
Observe for signs of pallor, nausea or light-headedness throughout the procedure.	To anticipate a syncope/ vasovagal reaction.
If the patient is sitting upright and symptoms become evident, place the patient's head between their legs and instruct them to take deep regular breaths.	To maintain patient safety.
If the venepuncture needle is in the patient's vein, complete the procedure obtaining the minimum amount of blood necessary to perform the required tests (if safe to do so). If unsafe, remove the blood collection bottles, release the tourniquet and remove the needle (venepuncture).	To avoid the patient having to undergo the procedure again. Removing the venepuncture needle reduces the potential of a needlestick injury occurring.
If appropriate secure the cannula in the patient's vein, if unsafe remove the device (cannulation).	A patent cannula may be needed to treat the patient.
Remain confident and calmly talk to the patient in a supportive manner	To provide reassurance.

Preventative action	Rationale
Document the incident.	To inform future practitioners about how the patient reacts to the procedure.
Stay with the patient until they feel well.	To ensure that the patient has time to discuss their reaction and is fully recovered.
Be aware that if the procedure is unsuccessful at the first attempt the patient may possibly become more anxious at the thought of a second attempt, causing vasoconstriction of their veins. Consider involving a more experienced practitioner.	The second attempt may be more difficult.
Advise the patient to inform all healthcare professionals about their reaction to needles/blood when they have the procedure undertaken in the future.	To ensure future practitioners can implement safety procedures.

NERVE INJURY

Extreme pain or numbness radiating down an arm is an indication that a nerve has come into contact with a needle (Boeson *et al.* 2000). The patient may complain of feeling an 'electric shock going down their arm'. Nerves are vulnerable to injury as they lie just below the skin in close proximity to veins, the two most commonly injured nerves being the radial and median nerves (Masoorli 2004). The radial nerve passes along the thumb side of the arm, from the shoulder to the wrist lying close to the cephalic vein, a site commonly chosen for venepuncture. The distal three inches of the radial nerve, just above the thumb, is most commonly injured during cannulation (Masoorli 2004). Cases have been reported of venepuncture performed at the anticubital fossa resulting in nerve damage affecting movement in the thumb and index finger many months after the venepuncture procedure (Zubairy 2002).

Specific precursors to nerve injury

- Poor site selection (Masoorli 2004).
- Inserting the needle too deeply into the tissue, or movement by the patient as the needle is inserted (McCall & Tankersley 2008).
- Blind probing with a needle when seeking a vein (Boeson *et al.* 2000).
- Haematoma formation, resulting in nerve compression (McCall & Tankersley 2008).

Prevention of nerve injury

Preventative action	Rationale
Practitioners must possess a sound knowledge of the anatomy and location of superficial nerves in the upper extremities.	To reduce the potential of piercing a nerve.
Avoid attempting vascular access on the inner aspect of the wrist.	To reduce the potential of damaging the radial, ulnar and/or median nerves located on the inner aspect of the wrist (Masoorli 2004).
If inserting a cannula into the cephalic vein, be conscious of the proximity of the superficial peripheral nerves (Boeson *et al.* 2000).	To reduce the potential of piercing a nerve.

Preventative action	**Rationale**
Palpate the vein of choice and ensure it is soft and bouncy.	To ensure it is a vein. Nerves are hard when palpated.
Prior to inserting the vascular device instruct the patient not to move their limb.	To avoid accidental contact with a nerve (McCall & Tankersley 2008).
Following insertion of the vascular device if blood is not visible in the blood bottle (venepuncture) or flashback evident in the chamber (cannulation) cease the procedure. Consider if techniques to correct missed vein entry (read 'Missed vein' section) can be employed or abort the procedure and begin again. Never probe blindly for a vein.	Blind probing is associated with nerve damage (Boeson *et al.* 2000).

Management of nerve injury

Action	**Rationale**
If an individual complains of an electric shock radiating down their arm, stop the procedure immediately and remove the vascular device as per local guidelines.	To minimise nerve damage. If the needle is inserted further, a permanent injury such as reflex sympathetic dystrophy (RSD) also known as complex regional pain syndrome (CRPS) may result. Symptoms include extreme sensitivity to touch and temperature, tissue swelling and pathological changes to bone and skin (Reflex Sympathetic Dystrophy Syndrome Association 2010).

Action	Rationale
Provide reassurance; explain why the pain/ numbness has occurred.	To reassure the patient.
Provide the patient with an information leaflet explaining what has occurred; discuss any concerns.	To reassure the patient.
Instruct the patient to contact a doctor if they become concerned about their symptoms, e.g. increasing pain.	Medical intervention may become necessary to treat the injury if it worsens.
If nerve damage is suspected, inform a doctor immediately.	Early recognition of nerve damage leads to a better patient prognosis and chance of recovery (Boeson et al. 2000).
Document the incident in the patient's notes.	To document the incident and assist with identifying improvement or deterioration of the injury.

ARTERIAL PUNCTURE

Arterial puncture is characterised by pain and the spurting of bright red blood out of an artery. Superficial radial arteries have been reported on the forearm lying close to the radial veins of the hand where they form the cephalic vein of the forearm (Rodriguez-Niedenfuhr et al. 2001). In this patient group it is possible to accidentally puncture the radial artery causing complications such as haematoma, temporary occlusion and pseudoaneurysm (Scheer et al. 2002). Inadvertent puncture of an artery is not uncommon.

Specific precursors to arterial puncture

- Morbid obesity, darkly pigmented skin or poor practitioner technique (Ghouri *et al.* 2002).
- Deep or blind probing, especially in the area of the basilic vein close to the brachial artery (McCall & Tankersley 2008).
- Failure to palpate a vein correctly (Lirk *et al.* 2004).
- Poor technique or assessment (Lavery & Ingram 2005).

Prevention of arterial puncture

Preventative action

If performing venepuncture or cannulation at the antecubital fossa or inner aspects of the wrist, palpate the site thoroughly prior to inserting a vascular device.

If it is difficult to distinguish a vein from an artery due to their close physical proximity, reposition the patient's limb and re-palpate the proposed puncture site.

Instruct the patient to keep their limb still while the vascular device is being inserted.

Rationale

To establish the absence/presence of a pulse. Pulses can be accurately detected by palpation. Only arteries have pulses. If a pulse is present identify another site.

To identify a suitable vein. This may take several attempts.

To prevent accidental puncture of an artery due to movement by the patient.

Management of arterial puncture

Action	Rationale
Arterial puncture can be recognised by bright red blood pulsing into the blood collection bottle (venepuncture), or pulsing out of the end of a cannula against gravity into the tubing of an infusion set (cannulation).	Signs that arterial puncture has occurred.
Remove the vascular device immediately as per local policy.	Incorrect structure has been accessed.
Apply digital pressure to the puncture site for 5 minutes (Lavery & Ingram 2005), elevating the arm to aid cessation of bleeding.	To stem bleeding (Dougherty 2008a).
Explain to the patient what has occurred.	To provide reassurance.
Do not reapply a tourniquet to the affected limb.	To prevent increasing vascular pressure and rebleeding at the puncture site (Dougherty 2008a).
Document the incident and provide the patient with contact details for whom to contact should they experience problems, e.g. numbness of the limb.	To comply with local reporting mechanisms (RCN 2010).
Provide information for the patient about what has occurred.	To provide reassurance.
Instruct the patient to contact a physician if tingling of their limb develops.	To ensure nerve compression has not developed as a result of continued bleeding.

PHLEBITIS

Phlebitis affects the inner endothelial layer of the vein (tunica intima). An inflammatory response is initiated as a consequence of damage to the endothelial cells which creates a roughened cell wall to which platelets readily adhere (Weinstein 2007). Phlebitis manifests itself as pain, oedema and erythema, typically presenting as a red streak along the length of the vein which can eventually cause the vein to feel like a cord (Macklin 2003). Phlebitis does not normally occur as a result of infection (Finlay 2004), but the site has the potential to become infected as a result of phlebitis. The two most common types of phlebitis are mechanical phlebitis and chemical phlebitis.

Pathophysiology of phlebitis

The moment a vein is punctured by a needle; damage occurs at the puncture site, and in some cases this will lead to the development of phlebitis. Damage at the puncture site causes the body's inflammatory response to be initiated, resulting in pain, redness (erythema), heat and swelling at the site. Damaged cells release histamine, bradykinin and serotonin. Histamine and bradykinin influence vasodilation, which increases permeability of the vein. Vasodilation encourages increased blood flow to the site of injury; increased permeability allows substances normally retained in the blood such as antibodies, phagocytes and procoagulant chemicals to be released at the injured site. Increased blood flow simultaneously removes toxins and dead cells from the injured site to encourage healing. Erythema and heat at the site develop as a consequence of increased blood flow to the area, delivering white blood cells necessary for tissue repair. Pain occurs in response to inflammation, and is sometimes the result of injury to nerve fibres, release of toxic chemicals from microorganisms, or pressure from oedema (Tortora & Derrickson 2009; Seeley *et al.* 2008). If the offending device is not removed from the body, leucocytes will accumulate at the inflamed site, resulting in further inflammation and eventually pus formation.

Specific predisposing factors for phlebitis

- Duration of time cannula has been in situ and type of infusate (Wilson 2008).

- Siting a large cannula in a small vein (Weinstein 2007).
- Poor positioning; over a joint or point of flexure (Finlay 2004).
- Cannula material: polytetrafluoroethylene (Teflon) is associated with more instances of phlebitis than polyurethane (Vialon) (Maki & Ringer 1991).
- Insufficient securing of the device (Finlay 2004).
- Gender: females are most commonly affected (Maki & Ringer 1991).
- Host factors, such as age and disease processes (Perucca 2010).
- Experiencing phlebitis on initial cannulation. This increases patient susceptibility on subsequent cannulations (Maki & Ringer 1991).
- Inappropriate administration of drugs, e.g. rapid infusion of fluids (Weinstein 2007).

Phlebitis scores

Phlebitis scoring systems, e.g. visual infusion phlebitis scores (VIP scores), assist practitioners to identify signs of phlebitis by measuring the most severe presenting complication against a standardised checklist (Jackson 1998; DH 2003). This enables the practitioner to decide whether the device is safe to be left in place, or should be removed and resited. The practitioner must inspect the cannula site a minimum of once per shift, each time a bolus infusion is administered, intravenous infusion rates altered or when intravenous solutions are renewed (RCN 2010). Using a scoring system encourages early detection of developing phlebitis and safeguards the patient's venous access for future use (Jackson 1998). Patients should be educated and encouraged to report changes to how their cannula looks or feels as they will often be the first to notice if a cannula is not working efficiently.

To use the VIP score the practitioner assesses the appearance of a cannula site and scores this against the phlebitis scale, e.g. a healthy site equates to stage 0 (see Fig. 8.1 for an example of a cannula care plan which uses a visual scoring system). If two of the following are evident: pain, erythema or swelling at the cannula site, then this equates to stage 2, at which point the cannula must be removed. If the cannula is to remain in situ beyond 72 hours then justification for the decision must be

Patient's name: ....   Hospital No: ....
Date of birth: ....   Ward ....

(Addressograph label may be used)

Need/problem
Intravenous cannula in situ for administration of drug therapy

Aim/Outcome
Cannula to remain patent and free from infection

VIP Score (VISUAL INFUSION PHLEBITIS SCORE)

OBSERVATION		ACTION
IV site appears healthy	**0**	No signs of phlebitis OBSERVE CANNULA each shift
One of the following is evident: Slight pain near IV site or slight redness near IV site	**1**	Possible first signs of phlebitis OBSERVE CANNULA
Two of the following are evident • Pain near IV site • Erythema - (redness) • Swelling	**2**	Early stage of phlebitis RESITE CANNULA
All of the following are evident: • Pain along path of cannula • Erythema (redness) • Hardening of tissue (Tissue feeling firm and swollen)	**3**	Medium stage of phlebitis RESITE CANNULA CONSIDER TREATMENT
All of the following are evident and extensive: • Pain along path of cannula • Palpable venous cord • Erythema • Hardening of tissue	**4**	Advanced stage of phlebitis or start of thrombophlebitis RESITE CANNULA CONSIDER TREATMENT
All of the following are evident and extensive: • Pain along path of cannula • Palpable venous cord • Erythema • Pyrexia • Hardening of tissue	**5**	Advanced stage of thrombophlebitis INITIATE TREATMENT RESITE CANNULA

Intravenous cannula care

1. Explain all procedures to patient/parent/carer
2. Cannula to be sited using aseptic technique
3. Document cannulation date, time, size, site, batch number
4. Examine and document the continuing need for the cannula on every shift and document 'Yes/No' in the appropriate boxes.
5. Inspect the cannula site on every shift and record the score using the VIP scale.
6. Inspect the cannula site whenever drugs are infused and when intravenous therapy is changed.
7. New infusion lines must be labelled with date and time of commencement
8. If the cannula was inserted during emergency conditions and asepsis cannot be guaranteed it should be removed after a new one is inserted.
9. Secure cannula with appropriate dressing and replace if it is soiled or loose. Document Yes/No in appropriate boxes
10. If cannula remaining in situ longer than 72 hours record risk assessment/rationale for this on VIP sheet and in patient's notes

Fig. 8.1 Example of peripheral intravenous cannulation care plan. Used with permission of Royal Berkshire NHS Foundation Trust.

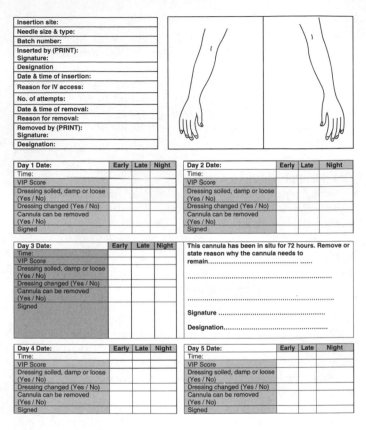

| Insertion site: |
| Needle size & type: |
| Batch number: |
| Inserted by (PRINT): Signature: |
| Designation |
| Date & time of insertion: |
| Reason for IV access: |
| No. of attempts: |
| Date & time of removal: |
| Reason for removal: |
| Removed by (PRINT): Signature: |
| Designation: |

Day 1 Date:	Early	Late	Night
Time:			
VIP Score			
Dressing soiled, damp or loose (Yes / No)			
Dressing changed (Yes / No)			
Cannula can be removed (Yes / No)			
Signed			

Day 2 Date:	Early	Late	Night
Time:			
VIP Score			
Dressing soiled, damp or loose (Yes / No)			
Dressing changed (Yes / No)			
Cannula can be removed (Yes / No)			
Signed			

Day 3 Date:	Early	Late	Night
Time:			
VIP Score			
Dressing soiled, damp or loose (Yes / No)			
Dressing changed (Yes / No)			
Cannula can be removed (Yes / No)			
Signed			

This cannula has been in situ for 72 hours. Remove or state reason why the cannula needs to remain.. ......

....

....

Signature ....

Designation...

Day 4 Date:	Early	Late	Night
Time:			
VIP Score			
Dressing soiled, damp or loose (Yes / No)			
Dressing changed (Yes / No)			
Cannula can be removed (Yes / No)			
Signed			

Day 5 Date:	Early	Late	Night
Time:			
VIP Score			
Dressing soiled, damp or loose (Yes / No)			
Dressing changed (Yes / No)			
Cannula can be removed (Yes / No)			
Signed			

Fig. 8.1 *Continued.*

clearly documented. Any incidence of phlebitis including intervention and treatment of the site should be documented in the nursing notes (RCN 2010).

Mechanical phlebitis
Mechanical phlebitis is associated with injury to the tunica intima from a cannula rubbing against the inside of the vein wall (Weinstein 2007).

Influencing factors
This is a problem commonly associated with inappropriate device selection and placement. Examples include placement of a large cannula into a small vein, or placement of cannulae near to joints or areas of flexion, causing the cannula to move in a piston-like manner, both practices resulting in damage to the tunica intima (Perucca 2010). Damage (pain, swelling, redness) can be observed at the cannula insertion site and/or along the side of the cannula stem.

Chemical phlebitis

Chemical phlebitis is associated with injury to the tunica intima by solutions infused into the venous system which cause inflammation (Weinstein 2007).

Influencing factors
Intravenous medications must maintain an optimum pH in order to work therapeutically; many drugs, however, deviate from the blood's normal pH level of 7.35–7.45 (slightly alkaline). Deviation from the blood's normal pH influences the development of chemical phlebitis. Normal pH of solutions is 7 (neutral). Solutions/medications that possess a high pH or osmolarity may predispose veins to irritation. The greater the acidity of a solution, the greater the potential for chemical phlebitis to develop (Perucca 2010). Damage to the vein (redness, swelling, pain) can be observed beginning directly at the tip of the cannula, extending up and along the length of the vein.

Prevention of mechanical and chemical phlebitis

Preventative action

Cannulae should not be left in situ if they are unnecessary and should not be sited for 'just in case purposes' unless clinical protocols dictate otherwise.

Rationale

To prevent phlebitis occurring in the first instance.

Preventative action	**Rationale**
Forward plan. Assess potential risk factors for medication to irritate the vein wall due to the pH or osmolarity (chemical phlebitis).	To assess if the patient would benefit from insertion of a CVAD, especially if drugs are to be infused over an extended period of time.
Contact pharmacy for advice.	To identify if it is possible to dilute the drug further, or decrease the rate of infusion to reduce venous irritation (Weinstein 2007) (chemical phlebitis).
Avoid cannulating areas of flexion or near bony prominences, e.g. antecubital fossa and inner wrist areas (Macklin 2003).	Cannulae sited near bony prominences may cause the patient discomfort and are associated with greater instances of mechanical phlebitis (Macklin 2003; Dougherty 2008a).
Avoid siting cannula in small superficial veins, e.g. the back of hands when infusing drugs with high pH or osmolarity (Finlay 2004).	Blood flow occurs more slowly in small peripheral veins, increasing the propensity for chemical phlebitis to develop (Weinstein 2007).
Avoid veins which are already bruised, painful, red, or feel cord-like when palpated.	These are unsuitable sites for cannulation as the veins are damaged and need time to heal.
Wherever possible avoid using the dominant limb.	The patient will use their dominant limb for the majority of activities; this increases the potential for mechanical phlebitis to occur if the cannula is sited in areas of flexion.

Preventative action	Rationale
Use the smallest gauge cannula capable of infusing the prescribed drug.	Smaller gauge cannulae are less likely to have contact between the cannula and the inside of the vein wall, reducing the potential for irritation of the inner vein wall (mechanical phlebitis) (Weinstein 2007). Smaller gauge cannulae encourage rapid dilution of drugs into the venous system (chemical phlebitis).
Wherever possible, avoid adding drugs via cannula injection ports or three-way taps.	Manipulation of cannulae during bolus infusions increases the potential for the device to rub against the vein wall, predisposing it to mechanical phlebitis. Three-way taps are associated with increased infection and phlebitis rates (Finlay 2004).
Consider the use of Luer lock design, needle-free add-on devices which allow the infusion of multiple drugs without manipulation of the cannula (in line with local policy).	Add-lines allow bolus infusions to be administered without excessive manipulation of the cannula.
After siting the cannula, secure it in place using an appropriate securement device and transparent vapour-permeable dressing.	To stabilise the cannula and allow easy inspection of the cannula site, encouraging early identification of mechanical/chemical phlebitis (Finlay 2004).
Rotate the cannula site every 72–96 hours or sooner, in line with local policy.	The longer the cannula is in situ the greater the potential for phlebitis to develop.

Preventative action

Use a standardised phlebitis scoring system to monitor and document the health of the cannula site (Jackson 1998).

Rationale

To prevent phlebitis occurring, remove the cannula when a VIP score of 2 is registered in line with local policy.

Consider the use of glyceryl trinitrate patches to promote venous dilation of small veins.

To expedite dilution of intravenous solutions into the bloodstream, reducing the potential for phlebitis to develop.

Management of mechanical and chemical phlebitis

Action

VIP score of 2 or more, remove the cannula in line with local policy.

Rationale

To encourage healing of the cannula site and prevent further damage to the vein.

A warm, moist compress may be applied to the affected site (Macklin 2003).

To reduce discomfort for the patient and improve blood flow to the affected area, thereby encouraging healing of the site (Macklin 2003).

Explain to the patient what has occurred and document the incident including removal of the cannula.

To document the incident (RCN 2010).

If the site is painful offer the patient simple analgesics.

To improve patient comfort.

If the infusion must continue where possible insert the new cannula into the opposite limb.

To rest the affected limb and encourage healing of the site.

Securement of cannula

Once sited it is important to secure the cannula in place to reduce movement which may cause migration of the catheter tip into surrounding tissue. This is especially important if individuals are confused or very young. The method of securement should not limit visual inspection of the insertion site, or interfere with the infusion flow rate (RCN 2010). Common cannula dressings include both gauze and tape, and transparent semipermeable polyurethane dressings. Both are non-occlusive, therefore preventing moisture collecting around the cannula insertion site. No statistical differences have been observed during comparisons between transparent dressings and sterile gauze (RCN 2010) but benefits and disadvantages of both types exist. Irrespective of which cannula dressing is used, they should be routinely changed each time the dressing becomes soiled or unsecured (RCN 2010).

Securement of administration set

To prevent the cannula from becoming dislodged or migrating from the insertion point, thereby increasing the potential for mechanical/chemical phlebitis, extravasation or infiltration to occur, it may be necessary to secure the administration set to the patient's skin. This can be achieved by creating a loop in the administration set tubing (being careful not to cause kinking of the set), then applying hypoallergenic tape firstly to the loop of the giving set and then to the patient's skin. It is important to avoid sticking the tape to the cannula dressing as this may reduce the moisture permeability rate of the dressing and inhibit observation of the insertion site. A careful assessment of the patient's skin integrity must be undertaken prior to use of tape, to ensure it will not precipitate skin tears.

INFILTRATION AND EXTRAVASATION

The words the 'drip has tissued' may be heard in reference to the leakage of therapeutic drugs into subcutaneous tissue as a result of a malfunctioning cannula. In reality what the healthcare professional is describing by this term is infiltration or extravasation; the outcome for the patient will be influenced by the incident that has occurred, and the actions taken to resolve the problem. Oncology/haematology patients are one at-risk group who often experience difficulties with venous access due to multiple punctures over long periods of time. Depleted venous access results in vascular devices being inserted into feet, the antecubital fossa or the back of hands, all sites at risk of infiltration/extravasation injury.

Specific predisposing factors of infiltration and extravasation

- Patients with poor venous access/fragile veins causing difficulties tolerating the volume, pressure or irritant nature of drugs (Dougherty 2008b).
- Poor positioning of cannula, e.g. near joints, back of hands (Finlay 2004).
- Peripheral neuropathy, decreased local blood flow, superior vena cava syndrome (Ener *et al.* 2004).
- Multiple punctures to the same vein or high infusion pressure (Schummer *et al.* 2005).
- Poor monitoring of the infusion (Dougherty 2008b)

Infiltration

Infiltration is the unintentional administration of non-vesicant drugs or solutions (drugs which do not irritate skin or veins) into the tissue surrounding a cannula, and is one of the most common complications of intravenous therapy (Weinstein 2007).

- Complete infiltration may occur as a result of a cannula being pulled out of a vein, or being forced through the vein wall on insertion (Lamb & Dougherty 2008).
- Partial infiltration may occur as a result of only the tip of the cannula being sited in a vein, or as a result of the vessel wall not sealing around a cannula tip, with the result that fluid slowly leaks into subcutaneous tissue (Lamb & Dougherty 2008).

Gravity then encourages the infusion solution to continue draining into the venous system. As a result, rather than fluid being transported via the venous system to the heart and body, fluid collects in the tissue immediately surrounding the displaced catheter tip. This flow will continue until interstitial pressure becomes greater than the gravity pressure of the infusate (Perucca 2010). Examples of non-vesicant solutions which may infiltrate include 0.9% sodium chlorate, and blood or blood products.

Patients experiencing infiltration may describe a cold sensation around the site of the displaced catheter tip, and the dressing holding the cannula in situ may become wet due to leakage of fluid from the puncture site. If a large amount of fluid becomes trapped in the subcutaneous tissue, the site may appear swollen, the skin shiny and stretched causing patient discomfort (Perucca 2010). Consequently infiltration may result in a reduction in the number of veins available for intravenous therapy due to oedema, and a risk of nerve damage or cellulitis to develop (Dougherty 2008b).

Extravasation

Extravasation is described as the inadvertent administration of vesicant drugs or solutions into the surrounding tissue instead of the intended vascular pathway (RCN 2010). Vesicant solutions when deposited into subcutaneous tissue have the potential to cause blistering and tissue damage which may lead to necrosis and damage to underlying tendons, nerves and blood vessels (Ener *et al.* 2004). Despite this, extravasation is generally underdiagnosed, underrated and underreported (Stanley 2002). The degree of damage caused by extravasation is influenced by the amount of the drug extravasated and the speed at which it is recognised. Signs of extravasation may not become apparent for several weeks, long after the patient may have been discharged from hospital. As a result, severe ulceration may develop unnoticed, leading to tissue sloughing and the necessity for skin grafting. Although uncommon, cases have been reported of patients undergoing limb amputation as a result of extravasation injury (Hadaway 2007). Examples of vesicant drugs include dopamine hydrochloride, norepinephrine, potassium chloride, amphotericin B, calcium, and sodium bicarbonate in high concentrations (Perucca 2010).

Pathophysiology

When extravasation occurs the patient may complain of burning or pain at the cannula site. It should be noted that extravasation can also occur without pain. Fluid leaks into surrounding tissues causing tissue compression as a result of the restricted blood flow; this reduces oxygen levels at the affected site, which in turn lowers the cellular pH. Capillary wall integrity is lost and oedema becomes evident, leading to tissue necrosis (Gabriel 2008). This process is influenced by the chemistry of the drug which has extravasated, and whether the drug binds to DNA. It is essential that clinical areas which administer such drugs have treatment protocols/policies in place so that staff are skilled to manage these incidents competently when they occur (Dougherty 2008b).

Prevention of infiltration

Preventative action

Rationale

Be aware of the vesicant potential of all infusions and medications.

To understand the risks associated with the drug.

Each cannula inserted should be placed above the old cannula site, preferably at least 3 inches (7.5 cm) above (Macklin 2003).

A new cannula sited below the site of a previous cannula increases the risk for development of infiltration.

Avoid siting cannulae near joints or bony prominences.

To prevent the cannula tip piercing the vein wall.

Use the smallest gauge cannula sufficient to infuse the intravenous therapy.

To encourage rapid dilution of the infusate.

Secure the cannula dressing and administration set securely.

To reduce movement of the vascular device.

Monitor infusions for signs of erratic flow. Check for resistance against the plunger when administering bolus drugs.

To detect possible signs of infiltration.

Preventative action

Do not force medications through a vascular device.

Winged infusion devices can be used to infuse non-vesicant drugs but are associated with greater instances of infiltration (RCN 2010).

Monitor the site regularly.

Rationale

Forcing infusions into a vascular device may precipitate infiltration

To encourage careful consideration of vascular devices available for infusing drugs.

To identify infiltration promptly.

Management of infiltration

Action

On recognition of infiltration discontinue the infusion immediately.

If in doubt that infiltration has occurred measure the girth of the affected limb then compare against the opposite limb. A simple visual assessment may be enough.

Remove the cannula and care for the site. If the solution is isotonic and has a normal pH, consider applying a warm compress to the affected area in line with local policy.

If the patient's hand/arm becomes swollen as a result of infiltration and they are wearing a ring/watch, remove them.

Explain what has occurred to the patient, inform medical staff.

Rationale

To prevent further fluid being infused into the patient's subcutaneous tissue.

To assess if the limb is swollen.

To reduce patient discomfort; encourage healing of the site and aid reabsorption of fluid by increasing venous circulation to the injured site (Perucca 2010).

To ensure that the swelling does not cause the ring/watch to become too tight, resulting in a diminished blood supply to the fingers.

To provide reassurance and make physicians aware of the incident.

Action	Rationale
Document the incident in the medical and nursing notes; include assessment of infiltration using an infiltration scale graded against the most severe presenting factor (INS 2006; RCN 2010). Where possible include photographic evidence.	To document the incident and assess the severity of the infiltration.
Infiltration statistics should be documented to include frequency, severity and type of infusate. Calculated as follows: (Number of infiltration incidents/Total number of peripheral IV devices) × 100 = % of peripheral infiltrations (Dougherty 2008a).	To establish how frequently this incident occurs.

Prevention of extravasation

Preventative action	Rationale
Ensure the healthcare facility has robust extravasation treatment policies/protocols and equipment available and staff are confident using them (RCN 2010).	To ensure that if an extravasation incident occurs the patient can be treated quickly using established policy.
Be aware of the vesicant potential of infusions and medications.	To identify potential risk factors.
Consider whether a CVAD should be inserted to infuse the medication.	To reduce the potential of extravasation occurring.

Preventative action	**Rationale**
Each cannula inserted should be placed above the old cannula site, preferably at least 3 inches (7.5 cm) above (Macklin 2003).	A new cannula sited below the site of a previous cannula increases the risk for development of extravasation.
If the patient has received multiple punctures identify their location, and establish how long ago the sites were used (Perucca 2010).	To avoid extravasation at sites distal to the cannula. Puncture sites not healed sufficiently have the potential to allow irritants to leak out of the puncture site into surrounding tissue.
Avoid cannulating beneath a recently punctured vein, e.g. after venepuncture.	To prevent irritant drugs leaking out of the puncture site.
Avoid siting cannulae near joints or bony prominences.	To prevent the cannula tip piercing the vein wall.
Avoid siting cannulae close to tendons, nerves or arteries; establish that the cannula is working correctly prior to use.	To reduce the potential for extravasation to occur, resulting in damage to essential vascular structures.
Wherever possible avoid using veins on the dorsum of the hand, in line with local policy.	Lack of subcutaneous tissue in the hand and close proximity to joints and tendons predisposes the patient to extravasation (Schummer *et al.* 2005).
Avoid siting cannula to infuse vesicant drugs, e.g. chemotherapy at the antecubital fossa.	Signs of extravasation may be more difficult to discern at this site, potentially resulting in damage to tendons, nerves and arteries (RCN 2010). To avoid damaging potential venepuncture sites.

Preventative action	**Rationale**
If possible use cannulae sited on the forearm to infuse vesicants.	Cannulae sited in the forearm experience less movement and can be securely held in place.
Infuse vesicant drugs first in a sequence of drugs.	To reduce the potential for extravasation to occur (Schummer *et al.* 2005).
Ideally use a newly inserted cannula to infuse vesicant drugs.	Vascular integrity deteriorates over time (Dougherty 2008b).
Use the smallest gauge cannula sufficient to infuse the intravenous therapy.	To encourage rapid dilution of the infusate.
Observe infusions for signs of erratic flow. Check for signs of resistance against the plunger when administering bolus drug.	To detect possible signs of extravasation.
Secure the cannula dressing and administration set securely.	To reduce movement of the vascular device.
Monitor the site regularly.	To identify extravasation promptly.
If a failed attempt is made to cannulate consider the possibility of using the opposite limb to site the cannula, in line with local policy.	To reduce the potential for extravasation to occur at old puncture sites (Gabriel 2008).
Do not use winged steel needles to infuse vesicant drugs.	Steel needles are associated with increased instances of extravasation.

Management of extravasation

Action	Rationale
Discontinue the infusion immediately.	To prevent further fluid being infused into the patient's subcutaneous tissue.
Implement the local organisation's extravasation policy/protocol.	To treat the site.
If appropriate leave the cannula in situ until blood and fluid has been aspirated and an antidote particular to the vesicant is instilled into the tissue in line with local policy (Perucca 2010).	To withdraw the extravasated drug from the infusion site and infuse an antidote.
Following removal of the cannula consider application of a cold compress to the site for alkylating and antibiotic vesicants; for vinca alkaloids consider application of a warm compress in line with local policy (Perucca 2010).	To treat the site.
Established policies/procedures must dictate the use of cold/warm compresses in line with local policy (Gabriel 2008).	Cold compresses cause vasoconstriction, localising the dispersal of the extravasated drug. Warm compresses cause vasodilation; beneficial for non-DNA binding drugs and applied after an antidote has been given. Increasing dispersal and absorption of the antidote into subcutaneous tissue (Gabriel 2008).

Action	Rationale
Explain what has occurred to the patient, inform medical staff.	To provide reassurance and make physicians aware of the incident.
Document in the medical and nursing notes the type of vesicant extravasated, amount infused, site of extravasation and the length of time the infusion had been running. Obtain photographic evidence if able. Adhere to local incident reporting policy.	To monitor the site.
Extravasation statistics (to include frequency, severity and type of infusate) should be collated by the healthcare facility using the green card system.	To document the incident. To establish incidences of extravasation locally and nationally. Incidences should be sent to: www. extravasation.org.uk.

INFECTION

Infection is more commonly associated with cannulation than venepuncture, although the potential does exist. As most cannulae are rotated every 72–96 hours if phlebitis develops it is usually of a mechanical/chemical rather than infective nature. Infection may be localised or systemic; localised infection is more commonly associated with cannulae. The pathogenesis of cannula-related infections is complex and carries the risk of systemic infection; if the patient is immunocompromised this may result in serious illness. Infection may result due to a number of predisposing factors.

Specific predisposing factors for infection

- Inadequate hand hygiene (WHO 2009).
- Re-palpation of a proposed puncture site immediately prior to introducing a device (Ernst 2001).

- Intrinsic and/or extrinsic contamination of therapeutic drugs, fluids or equipment used to treat patients (Finlay 2004).
- Use of contaminated tape to seal a puncture site (Weinstein 2007).
- Contamination of injection ports, hubs and bungs by microorganisms (Wilson 2008).
- Immunosuppression, loss of skin integrity, placement of multiple intravenous devices, age, genetics (Hart 2008).
- Skin organisms existing at the cannula insertion site migrating along the cannula track, or the cannula lumen, eventually colonising the cannula tip (Wilson 2008).
- Infection due to endogenous or exogenous pathogens (Hindley 2004).

Prevention of infection

Preventative action	Rationale
Always wash hands prior to performing venepuncture or cannulation or before manipulating infusion equipment.	Hand washing is a major infection prevention strategy (WHO 2009).
Screen patient's skin for skin commensals known to colonise intravenous devices, e.g. *Staphylococcus aureus*.	To identify which patients may require skin decolonisation.
Evaluate venepuncture/ cannulation equipment in association with procurement.	Cannulae with irregular surfaces readily become colonised by bacteria such as *Staphylococcus epidermidis*. Cannulae with smooth surfaces, e.g. Teflon or polyurethane, are more resistant to microbial colonisation (Sheth *et al.* 1983).

Preventative action	Rationale
Observe strict asepsis during the insertion procedure.	To prevent transfer of micro-organisms from the hands of practitioners onto the patient (RCN, 2010).
Insert intravenous cannulae using a sterile pack and aseptic technique.	To prevent microorganisms being inserted into the vein.
Use a fresh venepuncture needle/cannula for each attempt.	The venepuncture needle/ cannula will not be sterile or as sharp once it has punctured the skin.
Use appropriate skin decontaminants prior to accessing veins, i.e. 2% chlorhexidine, 70% alcohol (Pratt *et al.* 2007).	To decontaminate the skin prior to insertion of vascular devices.
Decontaminate the site for 30 seconds and allow 30 seconds for the agent to dry.	To decontaminate the skin.
Limit the number of attempts to insert a vascular device.	Skin puncture sites provide a route of entry for microorganisms (Hindley 2004).
Clip hairy limbs rather than shaving them prior to cannula insertion (RCN 2010).	To reduce the potential of causing micro-abrasions via which microorganisms can enter the bloodstream.
Avoid cannulating the lower extremities, i.e. femoral veins, unless unavoidable.	The lower extremities are associated with greater instances of infection (Parker 2002).
Assess the site using a visual scoring system such as the VIP score. Remove the cannula if VIP score >2 (cannulation) (Jackson 1998).	To prevent an infection occurring. Removal of the cannula will reduce the potential for a systemic infection to develop.

Preventative action	**Rationale**
Flush cannula sites regularly in line with local policy.	To prevent microorganims adhering to the cannula lumen.
Replace administration sets regularly in line with local policy (RCN 2010).	Bacteria introduced via contaminated infusates/ equipment multiply over time. Changing administration sets on a regular basis reduces the potential for contamination.
Ensure cannula dressings are applied correctly and removed when soiled.	To prevent moisture collecting under the dressing, allowing microorganisms to multiply.
Rotate cannula sites in line with local policy. Cannulae should be removed and the site rotated every 72–96 hours or sooner if problems are suspected (DH 2007).	The longer a cannula is in situ, the greater the potential for infection to develop.
All cannulae should be removed immediately on cessation of intravenous therapy.	Because they are no longer required to deliver intravenous therapy.
Peripheral cannulae inserted in an emergency should be replaced within 24 hours (RCN 2010).	Principles of asepsis may be compromised, potentially exposing the patient to infection.

Management of infection

Action	**Rationale**
The patient may complain of pain at the venepuncture/ cannula site. Investigate the area for signs of erythema, pain or swelling.	To identify an inflammatory response at the site.

Action	Rationale
Remove the vascular device (cannulation).	To prevent further discomfort and encourage healing of site.
Monitor the patient's vital signs for evidence of systemic infection.	To identify a developing infection.
If clinically indicated take blood cultures in line with local policy.	To identify if a bacteraemia has developed (Wilson 2008).
If infection is suspected or pus is evident at the cannula site, culture the cannula tip in line with local policy.	To identify if antibiotic therapy is required.
Apply a warm compress to the site.	To improve circulation to the affected area to encourage healing.

CONCLUSION

There are a number of factors to consider when attempting venepuncture and cannulation: correct technique, use of correct equipment, knowledge of anatomy and physiology and anticipation of potential complications. This chapter has identified the most common complications associated with venepuncture and cannulation with their predisposing factors and management. Understanding and employing these techniques will enable future practitioners to manage each complication competently and professionally as it arises in order to ensure the safety of their patients.

REFERENCES

Boeson, M.B., Hranchook, A. & Stoller, J. (2000) Peripheral nerve injury from a peripheral intravenous cannulation: a case report. *AANA Journal*, **69**(10), 53–57.

Campbell, H., Carrington, M. & Limber, C. (1999) A practical guide to venepuncture and management of complications. *British Journal of Nursing*, **8**(7), 426–431.

Collins, M. Phillips, S. Dougherty, L. de Verteuil, A. & Morris, W. (2006) A structured learning programme for venepuncture and cannulation. *Nursing Standard*, **20**(26), 34–40.

Deacon, B. & Abramowitz, J. (2006) Fear of needles and vasovagal reactions among phlebotomy patients. *Journal of Anxiety Disorders*, **20**(7), 946–960.

Department of Health (DH) (2001a) Consent – What you have a right to expect: A guide for adults. Available from: http://www.dh.gov.uk/en/Publicationsandstatistics/Publications/PublicationsPolicyAndGuidance/DH_4005204 (accessed 9 May 2009).

Department of Health (DH) (2001b) Good Practice in Consent Implementation Guide: Consent to Examination or Treatment. Available from: http://www.dh.gov.uk/en/Publicationsandstatistics/Publications/PublicationsPolicyAndGuidance/DH_4005762 (accessed 9 May 2009).

Department of Health (DH) (2003) *Winning Ways. Working together to reduce healthcare associated infection in England*. DH, London.

Department of Health (DH) (2007) *Saving Lives: High Impact Intervention No 2, Peripheral intravenous cannula care bundle*. DH, London.

Dimech, A. *et al.* (2011) Undertaking diagnostic tests In: *The Royal Marsden Hospital Manual of Clinical Nursing Procedures* (eds L. Dougherty & S. Lister), 8th edn. Wiley-Blackwell, Oxford.

Dougherty, L. (2008a) Obtaining peripheral venous access. In: *Intravenous Therapy in Nursing Practice* (eds L. Dougherty & J. Lamb), 2nd edn, pp. 225–270. Churchill Livingstone, Edinburgh.

Dougherty, L. (2008b) IV therapy: recognising the differences between infiltration and extravasation. *British Journal of Nursing*, **17**(14), 896–901.

Ener, R.A., Meglathery, S.B. & Styler, M. (2004) Extravasation of systemic hemato-oncological therapies. *Annals of Oncology*, **15**, 858–862.

Ernst, D.J. (2001) The right way to do blood cultures. *RN*, **64**(3), 28–31.

Ernst, D.J. (2005) *Applied Phlebotomy*. Lippincott Williams & Wilkins, Baltimore.

Finlay, T. (2004) *Intravenous Therapy*. Blackwell Publishing, Oxford.

Gabriel, J. (2008) –Safe handling and administration of intravenous cytotoxic drugs. In: *Intravenous Therapy in Nursing Practice* (eds L. Dougherty & J. Lamb), 2nd edn, pp. 461–494. Churchill Livingstone, Edinburgh.

Ghouri, A.F., Mading, W. & Prabaker, K. (2002) Accidental intra-arterial drug injections via intravascular catheters placed on the dorsum of the hand. *Anesthesia and Analgesia*, **95**, 487–491.

Hadaway, L. (2007) Infiltration and extravasation. *American Journal of Nursing*, **107**(8), 64–72.

Hart, S. (2008) Infection control in intravenous therapy. In: *Intravenous Therapy in Nursing Practice* (eds L. Dougherty & J. Lamb), 2nd edn, pp. 87–116. Churchill Livingstone. Edinburgh.

Hindley, G. (2004) Infection control in peripheral cannulae. *Nursing Standard*, **18**(27), 37–40.

Intravenous Nurses Society (INS) (2006) Infusion nursing standards of practice. *Journal of Infusion Nursing*, **29**(1), Supplement.

Jackson, A. (1998) A battle in vein against infusion phlebitis. *Nursing Times*, **94**(4), 68–71.

Lamb, J. & Dougherty, L. (2008) Local and systemic complications of intravenous therapy. In: *Intravenous Therapy in Nursing Practice* (eds L. Dougherty & J. Lamb), 2nd edn, pp. 167–196. Churchill Livingstone, Edinburgh.

Lavery, I. & Ingram, I. (2005) Venepuncture: best practice. *Nursing Standard*, **19**(49), 55–65.

Lirk, P., Keller, C., Colvin, J., Reider, J., Maurer, H. & Moriggl, B. (2004) Unintentional arterial puncture during cephalic vein cannulation case report and anatomical study. *British Journal of Anaesthesia*, **92**(5), 740–742.

Macklin, D. (2003) Phlebitis: a painful complication of peripheral IV catheterisation that may be prevented. *American Journal of Nursing*, **103**(2), 55–60.

Maki, D.G. & Ringer, M. (1991) Risk factors for infusion-related phlebitis with small peripheral venous catheters. A randomized controlled trial. *Annals of Internal Medicine*, **114**(10), 845–854.

Masoorli, S. (2004) Caution nerve injuries during venepuncture. Nursing spectrum. Available from http://community.nursingspectrum.com/MagazineArticles/article.cfm?AID=12773 (accessed 17 April 2009).

McCall, R.E. & Tankersley, C.M. (2003) *Phlebotomy Essentials*, 4th edn. Lippincott Williams & Wilkins, Philadelphia.

Morris, W. & Tay, M. (2008) Strategies for preventing peripheral intravenous cannula infection. *British Journal of Nursing*, **17**(19), S14–S21.

Ost, L. (1991) Acquisition of blood and infection phobia and anxiety response patterns in clinical patients. *Behaviour Research Therapy*, **29**, 323–331.

Parker, L. (2002) Management of intravascular devices to prevent infection. *British Journal of Nursing*, **11**(4), 240–246.

Perucca, R. (2010) Peripheral venous access devices. In: *Infusion Nursing: An evidence based approach* (eds M. Alexander, A. Corrigan, L. Goski, J. Hankins & R. Perucca), 3rd edn, 456–479. Saunders Elsevier, Philadelphia.

Pratt, R.J., Pellowe, C.M., Wilson, J.A., *et al.* (2007) epic2: National evidence-based guidelines for preventing healthcare-associated infections in NHS hospitals in England. *Journal of Hospital Infection*, **65**(Suppl. 1), S1–64.

Reflex Sympathetic Dystrophy Syndrome Association (2010) Available from: http://www.rsds.org/2/index.html (accessed 24 Nov 2010).

Rodriguez-Niedenfuhr, M., Vasquez, T., Nearn, L., Ferreira, B., Parkin, I. & Sannudo, J.R. (2001) Variations of the arterial pattern in the upper limb revisited: a morphological and statistical study with a review of the literature. *Journal of Anatomy*, **199**, 547–566.

RCN (2010) *Standards for Infusion Therapy*, 3rd edn. RCN, London.

Scales, K. (2005) Vascular access: a guide to peripheral venous cannulation. *Nursing Standard*, **19**(49), 48–52.

Scheer, B., Perel, A. & Pfeiffer, U.J. (2002) Clinical review: complications and risk factors of peripheral arterial catheters used for hemodynamic monitoring in anaesthesia and intensive care medicine. *Critical Care*, **6**(3), 198–204.

Schummer, W., Schummer, C., Bayer, O., Muller, A., Bredle, D. & Karzai, W. (2005) Extravasation injury in the perioperative setting. *Anaesthesia and Analgesia*, **100**, 722–727.

Seeley, R., Stephens, T. & Tate, P. (2008) *Anatomy and Physiology*, 8th edn. McGraw Hill International, New York.

Sheth, N.K., Rose, H.D., Franson, T.R., *et al* (1983) Colonisation of bacteria on polyvinyl chloride and Teflon catheters in hospitalised patients. *Journal of Clinical Microbiology*, **18**(5), 1061–1063.

Stanley, A. (2002) Managing complications of chemotherapy administration. In: *The Cytotoxics Handbook* (eds M.C. Allwood, P. Wright & A. Stanley), 4th edn, pp. 119–184. Radcliffe Medical Press, Oxford.

Tortora, G.J. & Derrickson, B. (2009) *Principles of Anatomy and Physiology*, 12th edn. John Wiley & Sons, Inc., USA.

Weinstein, S. M. (2007) *Plumer's Principles and Practice of Intravenous Therapy*, 8th edn, pp. 152–187. Lippincott Williams & Wilkins, Philadelphia.

Willemsen, H., Chowdhury, U. & Briscall, L. (2002) Needle phobia in children: a discussion of aetiology and treatment options. *Clinical Child Psychology and Psychiatry*, **7**(4), 609–619.

Wilson, J. (2008) *Clinical Microbiology: An Introduction for Healthcare Professionals*, 8th edn, pp. 307–350. Baillière Tindall, London.

WHO (2009) WHO *Guidelines on Hand Hygiene in Health Care First Global Patient Safety Challenge Clean Care is Safe Care*. WHO. Geneva. Available from http://whqlibdoc.who.int/publications/2009/9789241597906_eng.pdf (accessed 4 October 2010).

Zubairy, A. (2002) How safe if blood sampling? Anterior interosseus nerve injury by venepuncture. *Postgraduate Medical Journal*, **78**, 625.

Introduction to Routine Blood Tests, Normal Values and Relevance to Clinical Practice

9

Andrea Blay

LEARNING OUTCOMES

The practitioner will be able to:

❏ List the main blood tests and why they are indicated in particular patient groups.

❏ Identify patient factors to consider when taking blood.

❏ Understand the interpretation of the results within the clinical context.

❏ Identify technical problems to consider during the process of taking blood, e.g. haemolysis.

INTRODUCTION

Blood is the most studied tissue in the human body (Marieb & Hoehn 2007). In 2007/8 the NHS reported that £53.2 million was spent on testing over 9.1 million blood specimens (ISD 2008). Blood results provide valuable information on the biochemical and haematological functions of the body. When interpreted in the context of each clinical presentation they can reveal the presence of infections, genetic conditions and serious life-threatening

Venepuncture and Cannulation, first edition. Edited by Sarah Phillips, Mary Collins and Lisa Dougherty. Published 2011 by Blackwell Publishing Ltd.
© 2011 Blackwell Publishing Ltd.

diseases such as cancer. This chapter introduces the practitioner to the most common types of blood tests with examples of clinical application. Additionally, the tables provide a reference tool to aid practitioners in linking physiology to practical application and disease management.

WHAT IS THE PURPOSE OF TESTING THE BLOOD?

Blood testing is a fundamental part of the diagnostic process, providing essential information on which many clinical decisions and treatments are made. Blood tests confirm diagnosis and are also useful in eliminating other conditions which may have similar signs and symptoms.

The purpose of performing blood tests may fall into one of several catergories.

Blood grouping

A patient's blood group and antibody status must be checked prior to receiving a blood transfusion, blood products or before donating blood; and in addition human lymphocyte antigen (HLA) and tissue typing must be performed if undergoing organ donation or transplantation. Routine procedures and preoperative preparation should also include blood grouping and antibody status. Any patient undergoing surgery must have their blood group identified in case of major haemorrhage during or post procedure.

Testing for toxicity and illegal substances

Testing is done to ascertain if illegal drugs have been ingested or injected, as in a suicide attempt or accidental overdose to identify the nature and determine the amount of the drug taken. This is essential to establish the extent of the poisoning and may guide prognosis.

Some drugs, if allowed to accumulate to toxic levels or if they exceed their therapeutic range, can cause a variety of symptoms as well as resulting in renal impairment. They are commonly termed nephrotoxic, i.e. they have the ability to damage the nephrons, the functioning unit of the kidney leading to renal impairment or complete renal failure.

Therapeutic range

There are a number of drugs that have to be titrated to maintain certain levels to ensure that the drug is effective; this is the therapeutic drug range. Phenytoin, an anticonvulsant, is a good example: insufficient dosing can lead to fitting and loss of seizure control. Phenytoin has a narrow margin between therapeutic and toxic levels so monitoring of blood levels is crucial to avoid toxicity, which can manifest as nystagmus, ataxia, dysarthria, nausea, vomiting. If left untreated the patient may become unconscious and hypotensive, resulting in respiratory and circulatory arrest (Miller & Graham 2006).

The therapeutic range is assessed in relation to the following considerations:

- Physiological tolerance: Blood tests inform the clinician how well organs are functioning; the liver in particular is responsible for the breakdown and detoxification of many drugs. Likewise, the kidneys excrete the drug and its by-product. In liver and renal disease, toxins, the by-products of cellular metabolism and drugs, may accumulate and poison the body.
- Acceptable side effects: Some drugs can cause side effects which need to be monitored as well as monitoring the effects of the drug itself on the condition, e.g. an anticoagulant such as warfarin.

Infection and immunity

The microbiology laboratory undertakes serological, culture, sensitivity testing and direct microscopy to identify bacteria, fungi, parasites and ova (Bannister *et al.* 1996). Blood analysis of the white blood cells and immunoglobulins can help in understanding how efficiently the patient's defences or immune system are functioning and also determines the response to antibiotics or antivirals as well as monitoring the inflammatory response.

Blood is also tested to assess for a response to vaccinations, which provide an 'immunological memory' (DH 2006). This memory enables the immune system to recognise and respond rapidly on exposure to the antigen and at a later date modifying or preventing the disease. Antibodies can be detected in serum or plasma.

FACTORS THAT INFLUENCE BLOOD RESULTS

There are certain factors and variables that must be considered when interpreting blood results: firstly the environmental conditions of testing and secondly the patient or population demographics and medication profile.

Environmental conditions of testing

Table 9.1 summarises environmental factors that might affect the interpretation of blood results.

Patient demographics

- Biological variations within populations and between populations can influence the interpretation of blood results, e.g. race and gender.
- Endogenous substances can interfere with the laboratory result such as lipaemia, bilirubinaemia and paraproteinaemia (Knoll & Elin 1994).
- Increasing age should not affect blood levels despite functional and hormonal changes (Woodrow 2003a).
- Circadian rhythms, age, diet, caffeine consumption can also affect blood results (McCall & Tankersley 2008).
- Medications such as warfarin affect blood clotting (Reid *et al.* 2006). Potassium levels are affected by insulin (Reid *et al.* 2006). Inadvertent excessive potassium placement for patients on insulin therapy may have detrimental effects (see 'Biochemistry blood results' section). Some drugs have a synergistic interaction with each other which can affect blood tests.

METHODS USED TO OBTAIN SAMPLES OF BLOOD

There are several methods of obtaining a blood sample (see below), each of which is associated with technical factors that can affect the quality and accuracy of the blood results.

Blood can be obtained:

- by venepuncture when the vein is punctured solely for the purpose of withdrawing blood for testing
- from an existing intravenous device such as an arterial or central venous access device
- by capillary sampling
- from a peripheral cannula at the time of insertion.

Table 9.1 Environmental conditions

Factors that might affect the quality of the test and results	Rationale
Types of collecting tubes and sufficient additive present	Common additives include heparin, EDTA and citrate, which may affect ion-specific electrodes. The stoppers of some vacuumed specimen tubes are silicone coated and can affect the magnesium ion electrode (Knoll & Elin 1994)
The transport, storage and processing of samples. Vigorous mixing and/or exposure to extremes of temperature	Can cause cell lysis, affecting blood coagulation results (Lippi *et al.* 2006)
Prolonged tourniquet time	Tourniquet pressure and duration applied over 4–5 minutes can affect fibrinogen results by increasing the variability of the result (Rosenson *et al.* 1998)
Small or fragile veins requiring small gauge needles	Can destroy the red blood cell, causing haemolysis and providing erroneous results (Lippi *et al.* 2006)
Intravenous fluids such as 0.9% sodium chloride are known to be procoagulants Colloids such as Gelofusine and albumin also have significant anticoagulation properties	This affects fibrin formation, increasing coagulopathy (Coats *et al.* 2006)
Sample source: arterial, venous or capillary	There are slight variations in blood values obtained from different sources of vascular blood; it is important to note the source of the blood when documenting and interpreting results. Failure to do this could lead to misinterpretation, inappropriate treatments or lack of interventions

General points when obtaining a blood sample

1. As with all blood tests do not take blood from above the same vein that contains a cannula with an infusion in progress as this will contaminate blood results, especially when testing for electrolyte concentrations (see also Chapter 5).

2. The needle should not be too large because when blood is withdrawn too rapidly the red blood cells (RBCs) can rupture. K^+ and other ions can then leak out, giving a 'haemolysed' result or pseudohyperkalaemia (Perez 1995). Similarly, a large needle in a small vein will damage the vein needlessly (McCall & Tankersley 2008).

3. Using a needle with a gauge that is too small may cause haemolysis. Sizes range from 20- to 23-gauge and 21-gauge is considered standard for most situations (McCall & Tankersley 2008). (See also Chapter 5.)

4. Tissue damage can also cause K^+ to be released from damaged cells, e.g. prolonged application of a tourniquet (Lippi *et al.* 2006).

5. All tests should be repeated if the results appear spurious.

CLASSIFICATION AND MEASUREMENT OF BLOOD RESULTS

The different blood test tubes are separated once they reach the laboratory according to the blood test required into either haematology, biochemistry or microbiology departments (see Chapter 5).

For each blood test there are different units of measurement, and these should be checked against local references (normally noted next to the result) to detect for any variations from normal.

In the UK, blood tests are measured in Standard Units (SI) from the Système Internationale (SI) 1960 General Conference on Weights and Measures. This measures the number of moles per unit volume. The reference range for blood tests may vary from laboratory to laboratory and machine to machine. There are common normal values but the reference ranges provided by each institution are the ones to utilise in local clinical practice.

HAEMATOLOGY

Haematology is the study of blood and its components; this includes red and white blood cells, platelets and clotting factors. The heaviest and densest mass, comprising 45% of the total volume, is made up of red blood cells or erythrocytes giving blood its characteristic red colour (Marieb & Hoehn 2007).

Plasma is a less dense, straw-coloured liquid which constitutes about 55% of whole blood. Leucocytes or white blood cells and platelets (thrombocytes) comprise less than 1% of the total volume (see Chapter 1). The ability of blood to coagulate or produce a clot or thrombus is important in controlling haemorrhage. Clotting factors such as platelets and fibrin are utilised to form the clot and reduce blood loss. In some patients the blood has an over-tendency to clot, forming thrombi in the deep veins called deep vein thrombosis (DVT). The constituents of blood are prone to many diseases, such as anaemia, leukaemia and sickle cell disease, leading to derangements in the normal blood profile (Blann 2007).

A haematology service provides two main functions: (a) blood analysis and (b) the preparation and provision of blood and blood products for transfusion. Additionally, haematologists offer guidance on blood and diseases such as leukaemia and the haemoglobinopathies.

ORDERING HAEMATOLOGY BLOOD TESTS

The collective term for ordering blood tests for a haematological assay is a full blood count (FBC). The FBC is comprised of the red and white cell counts, differentials and the platelets. Assays of red blood cells (erythrocytes) include haemoglobin (Hb) and red blood cell indices which provide information on the size of the red cell, its mass and the overall available blood pool.

Red cell indices (see Table 9.2) include the mean cell volume (MCV), the mean cell haemoglobin (MCH) and the mean cell haemoglobin concentration (MCHC).

HAEMATOLOGY BLOOD TESTS

Haemoglobin

The main function of haemoglobin is to transport oxygen from the lungs to the tissues; the haemoglobin test provides information on the oxygen-carrying capacity of the blood. Therefore the purpose of performing a haemoglobin (Hb) test is to test for anaemia and/or polycythaemia, an excess red cell mass. The FBC also provides information on the size of the RBC, which is

---

> **Box 9.1 Clinical context – hypoxia and RBC production**
>
> Erythropoietin is an essential component manufactured by the kidneys in response to low oxygen levels; its function is to influence red cell production by the bone marrow. In chronic renal failure the kidneys are unable to produce erythropoietin, which affects red cell production. In hypoxic states the oxygen-carrying capacity of the RBC is reduced. In the critically ill, erythropoietin production is reduced due to low secretion by the kidney, which is exacerbated in liver and renal failure (Marieb 2006).

normally normocytic, and the colour – whether it is normochromic (normal colour) or hypochromic (pale colour).

The size and shape of the RBC are important in identifying diseases such as sickle cell anaemia and thalassaemia (collectively called the haemoglobinopathies). These are genetically inherited diseases found in specific patient populations. The red blood cells are significantly altered in shape and size and hence oxygen-carrying capacity is reduced in hypoxaemic states such as during exercise and when oxygen delivery and consumption is impaired such as in severe infections (see Box 9.1 and Table 9.2).

White blood count

The white blood count (WBC) or white cell count (WCC) blood test identifies the presence of infection or inflammation and provides an assessment of the body's immune response (see Box 9.2).

White blood cells are composed of different cellular components which are stimulated at different times and in different circumstances, their main function is to engulf and destroy microorganisms.

If the white blood cells or leucocytes have been stimulated this will cause a rise in the WCC and is a good indicator that the natural defences have been breached by invading microorganisms (see Table 9.2).

White blood cells exist in five different proportions; this is known as the white cell differential and comprises neutrophils, lymphocytes, monocytes, eosinophils and basophils (see Table 9.2). Neutrophils are the most abundant leucocytes, while basophils make up only 1% of the WCC (Blann 2007).

Table 9.2 Full blood count tests

Blood (serum) test	Normal values	Clinical application	Abnormal low levels and manifestations	Abnormal high levels and manifestations
Haemoglobin (Hb) Measured in grams per decilitre (g/dL)	Male 13.3–16.7 g/dL Female 11.8–14.8 g/dL White people have a slightly elevated Hb level by 0.7 g/dL (Rempher & Little 2004)	Anaemia is present when the Hb is less than defined normal values for gender and a low haematocrit Hydration can affect the Hb level: dehydration causes an elevated Hb; Over-hydration can lower the Hb level	The underlying causes for a low haemoglobin level are multi-factorial; in brief the aetiology of a low haemoglobin might be related to: 1. Red bone marrow dysfunction caused by cancer (acute and chronic leukaemia) 2. Active bleeding or haemorrhage from either external injuries due to trauma or internal bleeding from a ruptured aneurysm or gastric ulcer 3. Destruction of the RBC – haemolytic anaemia or cell lysis caused by incompatible blood transfusion and infections 4. Liver disease 5. Iron deficiency anaemia caused by malnutrition or poor nutritional intake of iron, folic acid and other essential minerals 6. Pernicious anaemia caused by vitamin B_{12} and intrinsic factor deficiency 7. Aplastic anaemia or bone marrow failure affects the production of normal RBC, WBC and platelets 8. Pregnancy Anaemic patients are often fatigued, pale and can be short of breath	1. Haemosiderosis (iron deposits in the tissues) (Andrews 1999) 2. Haemochromatosis 3. Polycythaemia (excess erythrocytes). The excess production of red blood cells can cause a number of problems; increased blood viscosity, which reduces fluidity of blood flow, causing stasis and increasing the risk of a stroke. In polycythaemia viscosity is increased, which causes blood to flow sluggishly (Marieb & Hoehn 2007) causing the haematocrit to rise, affecting the circulation and leading to fluid overload

Cont.

Table 9.2 Continued

Blood (serum) test	Normal values	Clinical application	Abnormal low levels and manifestations	Abnormal high levels and manifestations
Red blood cell count (RBCC)	Male 4.32–5.66 × 10^{12}/L Female 3.88–4.99 × 10^{12}/L		Decreased RBCC levels maybe due to haemorrhage and over-hydration	Increased erythrocyte levels maybe due to polycythaemia and dehydration
Mean cell volume (MCV)	80–98fL (femtolitres or 10^{-15})	MCV is the weight of the RBC	Microcytic anaemia or small sized RBCs are indicative of iron deficient anaemia and haemoglobinopathies	Macrocytic or large RBCs are seen in B$_{12}$ deficiency, alcoholism, hyperthyroidism, vitamin C deficiency and chronic liver failure (Elias & Hawkins 1985)
Mean cell haemoglobin (MCH)	27–34pg (picograms) or approx 640 million Hb molecules (Montague 2005)	Average mass of haemoglobin or the average weight of the RBC	Low MCH is associated with iron deficiency anaemia, thalassaemia, folic acid deficiency	Pernicious anaemia inc'eases the MCH (Rempher & Little 2004)
Mean cell haemoglobin concentration (MCHC)	20–35g/dL or 320g/L	Mean concentration of Hb in RBC	Low values due to iron deficiency anaemia, thalassaemia	Raised values due to intravascular haemolysis

Cont.

Erythrocyte sedimentation rate (ESR)	<10 mm/hour	See Blann (2007) for a description of how the ESR is obtained	Decreased ESR due to steroids, heart failure	There are many causative factors for a raised ESR: inflammation, tuberculosis, cancer, rheumatoid arthritis, inflammatory bowel disease. It suggests an acute phase response to infection or disease
Haematocrit (Hct) or packed cell volume (PCV)	Men 40–52% Female 36–48%	Hct the proportion of packed cells in a blood sample; this indicates the red cell mass relative to total blood volume (Montague 2005). Hct is a good indicator of the available RBCs within the blood pool	Low Hct: blood loss, over-hydration, anaemia	Increased Hct: dehydration, polycythaemia, chronic hypoxia (high altitude)

Table 9.2 Continued

Blood (serum) test	Normal values	Clinical application	Abnormal low levels and manifestations	Abnormal high levels and manifestations	Interventions
White cell or blood count (WCC or WBC) White blood cell count differential	3.7–9.5 × 10⁹/L or 4000–11 000/mcL Neutrophils 1.7–6.1 × 10⁹/L (40–50%) Lymphocytes 1.0–3.2 (20–45%) Monocytes 0.2–0.6 (2–10%) Eosinophils 0.03–0.46 (1–6%) Basophils 0.02–0.09 (<1%)	A normal physiological response to infection is temperature; older patients may present abnormal signs and symptoms of infection (Parker 2002; Watson 2000); therefore the WBCC is useful in determining whether infection is present in the elderly (Woodrow 2003a)	WBC count <3.7 × 10⁹/L is called leucopenia caused by typhoid, viral infections and leukaemia Neutropenia is a decrease in neutrophil levels; chemotherapy is another cause and this leaves the patient vulnerable to opportunistic infections or neutropenic sepsis	Leucocytosis or WBC >11 × 10⁹/L Autoimmune diseases such as arthritis can also stimulate the inflammatory response and increase the WBC levels Bacterial infections such as meningitis or pneumonia or bowel perforation cause the WBC to rise rapidly above 4000–11 000/mcL	Once antibiotic therapy has been introduced the WBC should be taken daily and in some instances more frequently to assess the body's response to the therapy. If the appropriate antibiotics have been selected the WBC should begin to decline. In cases of very severe infections the WBC may even decrease as bone marrow failure occurs

| Platelets (PLT) | 150000 to 400000/mm^3
The platelet count is the number of platelets in a blood sample | The platelet count is a useful diagnostic test when investigating abnormal bruising or an increased tendency to bleed due to other pathologies, e.g. aplastic anaemia
Platelets circulate and survey the endothelial lining of all cells, checking for cellular damage | Severe sepsis, cancer, portal hypertension, alcoholism and clotting disorders can cause a low platelet count or thrombocytopenia.
Thrombocytopenia can also be caused by some medications, e.g. heparin, rifampicin, digoxin, vancomycin. Antibodies can destroy platelets; failure of the bone marrow to produce platelets and increased consumption due to hypercoagulopathy states as seen in disseminated intravascular coagulation (DIC) can reduce the platelet pool (Rempher & Little 2004)
Massive transfusion or blood loss causes consumption of platelets and low platelet counts
Platelet counts of <50000/mm^3 may cause spontaneous bleeding (Rempher & Little 2004) | Raised platelet counts may indicate that infection is present | Platelet replacement is dependent on whether there is still active bleeding, resolution of the cause of the thrombocytopenia, ongoing cardiovascular instability and in bone marrow failure when the platelet count is <10000 or if the patient is undergoing surgery (Isbister 2003) |

> **Box 9.2   Clinical context – counting cells**
>
> **WBC counts**
> Neutrophils and macrophages are often referred to as 'cell eating' because they clump together around sites of inflammation so that their cytoplasmic enzymes can digest the engulfed microorganisms (Marieb & Hoehn 2007). Sometimes in acutely ill patients the neutrophil reserves may become so depleted that a neutropenia may develop rendering the patient susceptible to other infections. It is a sign of serious illness. Chemotherapy can also induce a neutropenia.
>
> **Platelet count**
> Platelets or thrombocytes are also part of the FBC test. Platelets play a vital role in controlling bleeding by producing a platelet or thrombus plug to achieve haemostasis.
> Platelets are analysed within the context of bleeding; if severe and prolonged bleeding is experienced the platelet count will fall as platelets are consumed in an attempt to maintain haemostasis (see Table 9.2). A reduced platelet count may lead to purpura, bruising and severe haemorrhage.

Blood clotting results

A clotting profile is undertaken to provide a haemostatic assessment (Isbister 2003), it includes the prothrombin time (PT), the activated partial thromboplastin time (APTT), fibrinogen and D-dimer assays (see Table 9.3). The PT and APTT measure the time it takes for blood to clot or form a fibrin plug at the site of bleeding; the endpoint of the coagulation system.

The coagulation system is a complex series of activators, inhibitors, factors and proteins that make up the extrinsic and intrinsic pathways. Blood is mixed with different activators to test the functioning of the extrinsic and intrinsic pathways (Higgins 1997). The prothrombin time is an assessment of the extrinsic pathway and the partial thromboplastin time or APTT tests the integrity of the intrinsic pathway (Hambley 1995) (see Box 9.3).

The PT is expressed as a mathematical equation known as the international normalised ratio or (INR). This is a standardised thromboplastin agent adopted by the World Health Organisation to reduce variability, improve reporting and assist in the management of warfarin therapy (Rempher & Little 2004).

Table 9.3 Blood clotting results

Blood (serum) test	Normal values	Clinical application	Abnormal low levels and manifestations	Abnormal high levels and manifestations	Interventions
Prothrombin time (PT)	11–15 seconds A control is used at the same time as the patient's results which are then interpreted against the control (Minors 2001)		Decreased levels due to blood clots, birth control medication	Prolonged in vitamin deficiency, liver disease, obstructive jaundice and intravascular disseminated coagulation (DIC) (McLaren 2005)	Observation of the patient with a deranged clotting should include assessing for signs of bleeding from the mouth and gums, haematuria (blood in the urine), gastric bleeding, bleeding from the bowel and increased tendency to bruise easily
Partial thromboplastin time (PTT) or activated PPT (APTT)	24–34 seconds	Affected by heparin		Prolonged in DIC, sepsis and liver disease Various factor deficiencies, e.g. factor VIII deficiency is a genetically acquired disease causing severe bleeding or haemophilia A Massive blood transfusion	Heparin, an intravenous or subcutaneous anticoagulant, prolongs the PTT/APTT
Thrombin time (TT)	10–13 seconds			DIC and liver disease increases the thrombin time	

Cont.

Table 9.3 *Continued*

Blood (serum) test	Normal values	Clinical application	Abnormal low levels and manifestations	Abnormal high levels and manifestations	Interventions
International normalised ratio (INR)	Target range 2–3 DVT, atrial fibrillation) 3–4 (post mechanical valve replacement)	The INR is used to guide and control warfarin therapy			The antidote to warfarin is vitamin K administered orally or intravenously In times of a clinical emergency, e.g. the need for an urgent operation, or gastrointestinal bleed, fresh frozen plasma (FFP) is given to reverse the effects of Warfarin
Fibrinogen	1.5–4 g/L or 200–400 mg/dL		<1.5 g/L – DIC Liver disease	>4 g/L sepsis, pregnancy, systematic inflammatory response syndrome (SIRS)	
D-dimers	<400–500 ng/mL (nanograms)	Measures the breakdown of fibrin		Often difficult to interpret in the presence of sepsis, post surgery or myocardial infarction when trying to diagnose pulmonary embolism and DVT as all of the above will elevate the D-dimer level DIC elevates the D-dimer level	

Box 9.3 Clinical context – activation of the coagulation system

The coagulation system is triggered by a number of mechanisms, and includes the complement, inflammation and immune systems. The exposure of damaged tissue to tissue factor activates the extrinsic pathway. Activation of the intrinsic pathway is via the contact phase and involves factors XII and XI.

Liver disease and vitamin K deficiency will affect the activation of the normal coagulation pathway leading to a prolonged prothrombin time and increase the risk of bleeding (Montague 2005).

Correction of coagulation disorders involves testing for congenital defects such as haemophilia A (lack of factor VIII) or Von Willebrand's disease. Other causes of haemostatic failure are massive blood transfusion, liver disease and disseminated intravascular coagulation (DIC), a complex coagulopathy often triggered by sepsis, massive trauma and endothelial wall injury (Levi & Cate 1999).

Replacement products include fresh frozen plasma (FFP), which contains clotting factors, and cryoprecipitate, contains factor VIII and fibrinogen (McClelland 2007).

The production of fibrinogen, a soluble protein, is essential to control bleeding; this is achieved by the activation of thrombin causing the soluble fibrinogen to become the insoluble fibrin (Breen 2004) to achieve haemostasis.

A D-dimer assay measures fragments cleaved from the activity of fibrin. The D-dimer test is specific for fibrinolysis, which is the breakdown and removal of fibrin once bleeding is controlled from blood vessels by enzymes and activators (Isbister 2003).

The liver produces many clotting factors some of which are dependent on vitamin K; these include prothrombin, factor VII and factors IX and X (Smith 2005b). Vitamin K is a fat-soluble vitamin; its own absorption is reliant on normal bile salt functioning and any reduction in bile flow will affect vitamin K absorption and availability to influence the production of clotting products (Smith 2005a).

Blood grouping and save and cross match

Prior to the administration of a blood transfusion the universal ABO blood group and rhesus (Rh) factor must be determined. The ABO system consists of four main blood groups: A, B, AB and O. Everyone is also either Rh D negative or Rh D positive (NBS 2008).

Group and save

A group and save is taken in advance in order to determine the patient's ABO and Rh D group. This enables any atypical antibodies to be identified as well as checking the results against any historical data that might be available for the patient (NBS 2008).

The *Handbook of Transfusion Medicine* (McLelland 2007, p. 16) advises that 'if red cells of an incompatible ABO group are transfused (and especially if a group O recipient is transfused with group A, B and AB red cells), the recipient's IgM anti-A, anti-B and anti-AB bind to the transfused red cells'.

Clinically significant antibodies are those that are capable of causing a transfusion reaction due to accelerated destruction of a significant proportion of transfused red cells. Anti-A and anti-B antibodies must always be regarded as clinically significant (NBS, 2008).

A blood sample will be referred to a red cell reference laboratory if there is any doubt concerning the identities of any antibodies present or lack of exclusion of clinically significant antibodies (Chapman *et al.* 2004). Failure to recognise all of the antibody specificities within a sample may lead to a haemolytic transfusion reaction (Chapman *et al.* 2004).

Cross match

Cross match will be performed to determine if the unit of blood is compatible with the blood of the intended recipient. This involves a serological test to ensure compatibility between a unit of blood and the patient (NBS 2008). Contreras and Mijovic (2009) state that it is mandatory to test the patient on at least two occasions before blood is issued in order to be certain of the patient's ABO group.

BIOCHEMISTRY

Biochemistry is the study of the biological and chemical compounds produced by organs and cellular processes. A biochemical assay may be performed for numerous clinical reasons ranging from assessing hydration status and electrolyte levels to monitoring specific organ functions of the liver, kidneys, thyroid and cardiovascular system, as well as the endocrine and

Table 9.4 Ordering biochemistry blood tests

Blood test	Components
U&Es: urea and electrolytes	Sodium (Na$^+$), potassium (K$^+$), urea (Ur) and creatinine (Cr)
Liver function tests (LFTs) and protein assays	Bilirubin, alanine aminotransferase (ALT), alkaline phosphatase (ALP) and aspartate aminotransferase (AST) Protein measurements such as albumin, total protein and globulin
Bone profile	Calcium (Ca^{2+}) and phosphate (PO$_4^-$)
Cardiac and thyroid function	Troponin Lactate dehydrogenase (LDH) Cholesterol Fasting blood glucose Thyroid stimulating hormone, parathyroid and thyroid hormones
Acute phase proteins	C-reactive protein (CRP)
Additional biochemistry tests	Magnesium (Mg^{2+}) Lactate Amylase

hormonal systems. Biochemistry results can also provide valuable information on the status of diseases such as diabetes, hyperlipidaemia, atherosclerosis and infections (see Table 9.4).

Other blood tests specific for certain markers of disease are not included in this chapter, such as human immunodeficiency virus (HIV), cancer tumour markers and immunoglobulins (e.g. IgM, IgA, IgG) made by B lymphocytes and released as part of the humoral response to infection and pathogens.

BIOCHEMISTRY BLOOD RESULTS

Urea and electrolytes (see Table 9.5)

Electrolytes

Blood or serum tests measure the concentration of electrolytes and other solutes in the plasma or the extracellular fluid (ECF)

Table 9.5 Urea and electrolyte values

Blood (serum) test	Normal values	Clinical application	Abnormal low levels and manifestations	Abnormal high levels and manifestations	Interventions
Sodium (Na⁺) test Serum sodium is a common blood test performed to ascertain fluid status and the need for water (Sterns & Silver 2003) It is the main cation in blood and extracellular fluid	135–145 mmol/L Intracellular Na⁺ level = 10 mmol/L	Assessment of hydration along with urea, glucose, skin turgor, thirst assessment, plasma and urine osmolarity levels and urine sodium levels (Patel 2007) Abnormalities in the sodium level may indicate a dysfunctional renal system as the main function of the kidney is to regulate water and sodium balance	Primary renal loss is mainly through diuretic therapy; other sodium losses occur with vomiting, gastric suction, pancreatitis, major burns and diabetic ketoacidosis (water moves out of the cell in hyperglycaemia). Excess water gain or hypervolaemia occurs from cardiac failure and cirrhosis (Criddle 2006; Reynolds *et al.* 2006) Clinical signs vary depending on the sodium level and how rapidly the sodium level has fallen; symptoms include malaise, nausea and vomiting Mild hyponatraemia (130–135 mmol/L) is often asymptomatic (Reynolds *et al.* 2006). Severe rapid onset of hyponatraemia can be a life-threatening condition leading to fitting, coma and death when levels fall below 110 mmol/L (Jamieson 1985).	Clinical signs: reduced skin turgor (unreliable assessment in older patients), sticky secretions and dry mucous membranes. Increased malaise and lethargy leading to coma Neurological signs include: disorientation, irritability, muscle twitching and seizures Haemodynamic signs: low urine output, tachycardia and hypotension Thirst is a late sign and not a good indicator of the severity of dehydration The plasma osmolarity and urea levels are raised in hypernatraemia	Accurate fluid balance charting is essential Careful restoration and attention to the rapidity of sodium and fluid replacement is required due to the risk of causing cerebral oedema

Blood (serum) test	Normal values	Clinical application	Abnormal low levels and manifestations	Abnormal high levels and manifestations	Interventions
Potassium (K⁺) Main intracellular cation	3.5–5.0 mmol/L Intracellular K⁺ level = 125 mmol/L	Changes in potassium concentration will affect the rate of depolarisation and repolarisation of the cardiac cell, ultimately affecting the heart rate and rhythm (Humphreys 2007). Potassium levels in cardiac patients should ideally be maintained >4.0–4.5 to prevent dysrhythmias (Jowett & Thompson 2003)	ECG features include: U waves, T wave flattening, ST segment changes, arrhythmias, cardiac arrest from VT/VF, asystole and PEA (Resuscitation Council 2010) Other clinical signs are fatigue, cramps, constipation and in severe hypokalaemia ascending paralysis leading to respiratory insufficiency (Resuscitation Council 2010)	Clinical signs include: slow and or irregular heart rate, muscle weakness, cramps and confusion Over 8 mmol/L: ascending paralysis can occur leading to respiratory arrest (Perez 1995) ECG changes induced by hyperkalaemia are complex and beyond the scope of this chapter; briefly there may be a missing or low amplitude P wave, peaked or tented T waves, widened QRS complex, shortened QT interval, ST segment changes leading to either asystole, ventricular tachycardia (VT), ventricular fibrillation (VF) and pulseless electrical activity (PEA) (Humphreys 2007; Resuscitation Council 2010; Holt 2008)	Treatment of hypokalaemia will involve sensible replacement of potassium whether orally or intravenously IV route: the infusion should be administered via an infusion device and in some cases the patient should be cardiac monitored Depending on the severity of hyperkalaemia, calcium resins may be considered, dextrose and insulin infusion, and in some cases the patient may need haemodialysis

Cont.

Table 9.5 *Continued*

Blood (serum) test	Normal values	Clinical application	Abnormal low levels and manifestations	Abnormal high levels and manifestations	Interventions
Blood urea nitrogen (BUN)	>2.5–8.9 mmol/L	BUN is taken to assess renal function, dehydration and fluid status	Malnutrition and advanced liver disease can reduce the urea level to below 2.5 mmol/L (Bratt-Wyton 1998)	Clinical signs of uraemia (high BUN level) are vomiting, diarrhoea and oedema. Cardiac instability can occur due to retained potassium leading to death (McLaren 2005) Urea is neurotoxic and may cause acute confusional states (Woodrow 2003b) Elevated BUN is indicative of a reduced circulating volume and reduced clearance of waste products. During periods of dehydration and hypovolaemia, aldosterone excretion increases sodium and water retention, reducing the GFR and causing the BUN levels to rise Other causative factors that will raise the BUN are vomiting, diarrhoea, infections and haemorrhage (McLaren 2005) A combination of a raised sodium and urea level are indicative of dehydration	Treating elevated BUN depends on the cause. Primarily a raised urea is associated with dehydration; the main intervention is fluid resuscitation to restore circulating volume In acute renal failure the main mechanism to reduce the urea is by haemofiltration In chronic renal failure haemodialysis and dietary control of sodium and protein are the cornerstones of treatment (NICE 2008)

Blood (serum) test	Normal values	Clinical application	Abnormal low levels and manifestations	Abnormal high levels and manifestations	Interventions
Creatinine	53–133 μmol/L	Specific marker of renal function	Increased water content increases its distribution thereby lowering serum creatinine levels Liver dysfunction and loss of muscle mass (Tillyard et al. 2005)	In critical illness interpretation of creatinine can be difficult as there are other factors that will raise the creatinine level including trauma, fever and immobilisation (Tillyard et al. 2005)	
Glomerular filtration rate (GFR)	GFR is normally 120 mL/min (McLaren 2005). GFR declines with age. Above 60 mL/min is acceptable	GFR is a very specific kidney function test. GFR is defined as the volume of plasma filtered in one minute by glomeruli (McLaren 2005). The GFR is calculated from the urine and serum creatinine level and 24-hour urine volume (Blann 2007).	Falling GFR indicates worsening renal failure		Drug doses should be reduced if the GFR is falling and in elderly patients due to declining GFR rates to prevent accumulation and nephrotoxicity

Cont.

Table 9.5 *Continued*

Blood (serum) test	Normal values	Clinical application	Abnormal low levels and manifestations	Abnormal high levels and manifestations	Interventions
Plasma osmolarity	280–300 mOsm/L Osmolarity is the concentration of moles in a litre. Primarily dependent on plasma concentration of sodium	To assess hydration status Plasma osmolarity is often performed along with urine osmolarity to exclude SIADH secretion	In hyponatraemia osmolarity falls	In cases of dehydration the plasma osmolarity increases; the thirst mechanism is triggered when plasma osmolarity is >290 mOsm/L (Vedig 2003) Osmolarity is increased in hyperglycaemia and elevated BUN states	

Blood (serum) test	Normal values	Clinical application	Abnormal low levels and manifestations	Abnormal high levels and manifestations	Interventions
Chloride (Cl⁻) anion	97–110 mmol/L	Routinely performed along with sodium	Hypochloraemia can be caused by vomiting and excessive sweating causing a metabolic alkalosis. It is also associated with hypokalaemia	Hyperchloraemia caused by the infusion of large volumes of 0.9% NaCl (saline) or ammonium chloride. Ammonium chloride 2.14% acid solution can be used to correct severe metabolic alkalosis (Metheny 2000) Diarrhoea due to the loss of bicarbonate salts can cause hyperchloraemic acidosis. Renal tubular acidosis associated with the loss of bicarbonate or inability to reclaim bicarbonate ions via the peritubular capillaries (McLaren 2005) Patients who have had a urinary diversion into the sigmoid colon or ileal segment lose bicarbonate in exchange for chloride (Metheny 2000) Hyperchloraemia may also affect coagulation as documented in aortic aneurysm surgery (Handy & Soni 2008)	0.9% sodium chloride contains 154 mmol of each ion and has been the mainstay of fluid resuscitation and maintenance regimens for the past 50 years (Handy & Soni 2008). The adverse effects of hyperchloraemia acidosis due to excessive use of saline are well documented; clinical side effects include changes in muscle contractility and reduced efficacy of inotropes (Handy & Soni 2008)

Cont.

247

Table 9.5 Continued

Blood (serum) test	Normal values	Clinical application	Abnormal low levels and manifestations	Abnormal high levels and manifestations	Interventions
Bicarbonate (HCO_3^-) anion	22–30 mmol/L	Clotted blood is required for the blood test	Clinical symptoms include headache, confusion, increased drowsiness, increased respiratory rate, nausea and vomiting. Causes include: diabetic ketoacidosis, lactic acidosis, liver and renal failure, lactic acidosis, poisons and toxin ingestion (Metheny 2000). Hypoperfusion and hypoxia can cause extracellular acidosis, resulting in profound cellular organ dysfunction (Handy & Soni 2008)	Causes: Loss of hydrochloric acid (HCl) from vomiting, nasogastric suctioning. Diuretic therapy causes hydrogen ion loss in the urine and excess reabsorption of HCO_3 by the kidney (Martin 1999). Administration of sodium bicarbonate and steroids. Severe K^+ depletion	Sodium bicarbonate is not routinely administered in cardiac arrest unless cardiac arrest is associated with hyperkalaemia or tricyclic overdose (Resuscitation Council 2010). Side effects of sodium bicarbonate infusion include rebound acidosis, hypernatreamia and hyperosmolarity

and not the intracellular fluid (ICF); this is technically difficult. Electrolytes acquire a positive (+) or negative (−) charge when dissolved in water.

Sodium, potassium, calcium and magnesium are examples of positively charged cations. Anions are negatively charged ions, e.g. chloride and bicarbonate.

Sodium (Na⁺)

Sodium is the most important and abundant electrolyte in the body intricately involved in the regulation of water content, and due to its osmotic action affects the plasma volume and blood pressure (Criddle 2006). Ninety-five per cent of sodium is found within the ECF. Sodium is lost from the body in sweat and during periods of dehydration from vomiting, excessive sweating and diarrhoea (Metheny 2000).

Any losses or gains in sodium will equate to a loss or increase in water content. Sodium chloride diffuses across a semipermeable membrane bringing about equilibrium in the sodium concentration. Simplistically wherever sodium goes water goes too (see Boxes 9.4, 9.5 and 9.6).

Potassium (K⁺)

Potassium is the most abundant intracellular cation (Worthley 2003); 98% is found within the cell (Metheny 2000). Potassium is constantly moving across the cellular membrane between the intra- and extracellular spaces (Humphreys 2007). It is important for maintaining muscle and nerve function during the transmission of nerve impulses. Potassium is mainly excreted by the kidneys; but some is lost from the gut during vomiting, diarrhoea and in sweat (Metheny 2000).

Conditions and interventions that can cause potassium shifts are trauma, tissue injury and shock, blood transfusion and insulin administration and rewarming after hypothermia (Edwards 2001). Both extremes of potassium imbalance; hypokalaemia and hyperkalaemia, can result in cardiac arrhythmias ventricular defibrillation and death (Resuscitation Council UK 2010) (see Boxes 9.7, 9.8 and 9.9).

Box 9.4   Clinical context – hyponatraemia or low sodium levels

A low serum sodium level less than 135 mmol/L is termed hyponatraemia or 'water intoxication'. It is the most common electrolyte abnormality (Fox & Fox 2007) and a common clinical finding, especially in older people (Holm *et al.* 2009; Woodrow 2003b). Premenopausal women seem to be particularly sensitive to hyponatraemia and the complications of cerebral oedema, especially in the postoperative period (Arieff 1993).

There are three main categories of hyponatraemia which depend on the precipitating problem: hypovolaemia as a result of extrarenal or renal losses; hypervolaemia or excessive extracellular fluid volume from congestive cardiac failure; and euvolaemia when the causative problem is not related to a lack or excess of fluid but from hormone deficiencies, e.g. pituitary and thyroid hormonal imbalances (Reynolds *et al.* 2006).

Aetiology of hyponatraemia

Hypovolaemia: loss of sodium

- Kidney disease – nephritis.
- Diuretics, e.g. thiazides.
- Adrenal insufficiency. Normally aldosterone influences the reabsorption of sodium and water. Adrenal insufficiency reduces the amount of aldosterone produced and sodium is lost from the renal system.
- Gastrointestinal losses, sweating and burns.

Hypervolaemia: water gains

- Oedema (cardiac failure and ascites).
- Nephrotic syndrome (Reynolds *et al.* 2006).

Euvolaemia

- Hypokalaemia – sodium shifts into the cell.
- Syndrome of inappropriate anti-diuretic hormone (SIADH) when too much anti-diuretic hormone (ADH) or vasopressin is released, causing excessive water retention. Global cerebral oedema can cause damage to the hypothalamus or pituitary gland, bringing about the inappropriate release of ADH increasing water loss.
- Head injuries, stroke.
- Pituitary tumours and other cancers.
- Respiratory diseases: pneumonia, asthma, tuberculosis.
- Compulsive water drinking (primary polydipsia), excessive administration of water or hypotonic fluids.

Pharmacological agents

- Non-steroidal anti-inflammatory drugs (NSAIDs).
- Omeprazole.
- Antidepressants, e.g. tricyclics (Metheny 2000).

Box 9.5   Clinical context – hypernatraemia or high sodium levels

Hypernatraemia is defined as a sodium level greater than 145mmol/L; it is much less common and associated with either water loss or sodium gain. Classification is according to the fluid states of hypovolaemia, hypervolaemia and euvolaemia (Reynolds *et al.* 2006).

Hypovolaemia
Increases in the sodium level have several aetiologies; the most common is insufficient oral intake, especially during periods of increased sweating, exercise and gastrointestinal losses. The elevated sodium level is caused by the excessive net loss of water causing an increased concentration of sodium in less water (see Table 9.5 for recognition signs and treatment). Other causes include diuretic therapy, acute and chronic renal disease and hyperosmolar non-ketotic coma).

Hypervolaemia
Excessive salt intake or sodium load from intravenous fluids such as mannitol (hypertonic solution) and sodium bicarbonate will raise the sodium level.

Euvolaemia
Endocrine and hormonal dysfunction such as diabetes insipidus causes excessive urine excretion (polyuria), which may exceed sufficient oral intake. In most people the thirst mechanism will drive the need for fluid replenishment and the sodium level will remain relatively normal. Other causes include fever and hyperventilation (Reynolds *et al.* 2006).

Box 9.6   Clinical context – heat stress

Salt depletion (hyponatraemia) from inadequate replacement of sodium in heat stress situations and during endurance events can cause heat exhaustion; additional symptoms include giddiness, diarrhoea, muscle cramps and headache (Anastasiou *et al.* 2009). This is different from heat exhaustion that is due to water depletion and resulting hypernatraemia (Metheny 2000).

Blood urea nitrogen (BUN)

Urea is the waste product of protein cellular metabolism (Marieb 2006). Forty to fifty per cent is reabsorbed from the filtrate, making it an unreliable test for assessing glomerular filtration rates (GFR); the rest is excreted in the urine (Traynor et al. 2006).

Box 9.7   Clinical context – hypokalaemia

Hypokalaemia is defined as potassium level <3.5 mmol/L. Severe hypokalae-mia is a potassium level <2.5 mmol/L. Loss of potassium may increase sus-ceptibility to ectopy and ventricular fibrillation (Jowett & Thompson 2003).

Aetiology of hypokalaemia

- Renal losses from the use of non-potassium-sparing diuretics, e.g. furosem-ide, a loop diuretic.
- Diabetes insipidus.
- Dialysis.
- Gastrointestinal losses.
- Metabolic alkalosis.
- Magnesium depletion.
- Reduced dietary intake.

Pharmacological agents that increase potassium loss are: salbutamol, dob-utamine, overdoses of verapamil and digoxin, a glycoside. Digoxin is used to control the heart rate, e.g. in atrial fibrillation. Hypokalaemia increases the toxicity of digoxin (Humphreys 2007).

Box 9.8   Clinical context – hyperkalaemia

The Resuscitation Council UK (2010) defines hyperkalaemia as mild elevation (5.5–5.9 mmol/L), moderate elevation 6.0–6.4 mmol/L and severe elevation >6.5 mmol/L.

Aetiology of hyperkalaemia

- Renal failure – acute and chronic due to decreased potassium excretion.
- Rapid IV replacement of potassium (>20 mmol/hour).
- Burns.
- Insulin deficiency.
- Acidosis.
- Diabetes mellitus.
- Diabetic ketoacidosis (DKA).
- Lack of aldosterone. Aldosterone causes retention of sodium and water. A lack of aldosterone causes retention of potassium (Wallace 2005).

Pharmacology agents

- Potassium sparing diuretics (e.g. spironolactone).
- Potassium supplements.
- Angiotensin–converting enzyme (ACE) inhibitors, e.g. lisinopril.
- Beta (β) blockers.
- NSAIDs especially in elderly people.
- Heparin (Metheny 2000).

Box 9.9 Clinical context – acid–base effects on potassium

Acid–base abnormalities are clinically significant when interpreting potassium levels because acid–base changes affect the cellular movement of potassium (Miller & Graham 2006).

Acidosis

In acidotic states when the pH is <7.35, potassium will leave the cell causing the serum potassium level to rise (Miller & Graham 2006); this can be life-threatening promoting the need for interventions such as the administration of glucose and insulin to reduce the harmful effects of elevated potassium levels (Mahoney *et al.* 2005). Correcting the acidosis reduces the serum potassium.

Alkalosis

A respiratory or metabolic alkalosis, when the pH is >7.45, will lower the serum potassium as the ions move back inside the cell (Jowett & Thompson 2003). Potassium movement is caused by hydrogen (acid) ions moving out of the cell to buffer the alkalosis (Miller & Graham 2006).

Insulin effects on potassium

Insulin therapy lowers serum potassium levels by increasing the cellular uptake of potassium (Edwards 2001); it is the main treatment for severe life-threatening hyperkalaemia. Conversely when insulin is being administered to control blood glucose, potassium levels should be monitored and replaced as required; otherwise the patient is at risk of the complications of hypokalaemia.

The BUN is unreliable as a measurement of kidney function (Stark 1994) as the daily urea levels are affected by the amount of dietary protein, gastrointestinal haemorrhage, surgery, tissue breakdown and steroid therapy, all of which increase urea levels (Traynor *et al.* 2006) making interpretation difficult.

Creatinine

Creatinine is the by-product of skeletal muscle metabolism; the daily amount produced is proportional to the body mass, which rarely changes (Marieb & Hoehn 2007) making it an ideal substance for measuring the GFR as creatinine is filtered by the glomerulus and is not reabsorbed (Traynor *et al.* 2006). Serum creatinine is proportional to the GFR, and may give an over-estimation of renal functioning (Tillyard *et al.* 2005). Creatinine

---

Box 9.10   Clinical context – chloride

Chloride reacts with HHb (hydrogen and haemoglobin) to release or unload
oxygen from haemoglobin into the cells. One chloride ion enters the RBC as
one bicarbonate ion leaves, which is known as the 'chloride shift' (Marieb &
Hoehn 2007). Chloride is excreted via the kidney, in sweat and in gastric acid.

---

is useful in highlighting deteriorating renal function, but the
trend is more helpful in monitoring the presence and progression of acute renal failure (ARF) (Tillyard *et al.* 2005). The GFR
is important in assessing the kidney's ability to excrete pharmacological agents (see Table 9.5).

Chloride
Chloride ion is found within the RBC, along with sodium and
bicarbonate; the three ions contribute towards the highest blood
concentration and electrical charge (Holum 1998). Chloride has
several important biochemical roles: it helps to maintain osmotic
pressure and fluid distribution, acid–base balance and oxygen
transport (Holum 1998) (see Box 9.10).

Bicarbonate
Bicarbonate is the main acid blood buffer forming the
bicarbonate–carbonic buffering system, in which acids are buffered and eliminated from the body. Carbon dioxide (CO_2), a
by-product of cellular respiration, is dissolved in water to form
the weak carbonic acid (H_2CO_3); it is transported via the red
blood cells to the lungs for excretion. Another term for bicarbonate is base or alkali (see Box 9.11).

Liver function tests (see Table 9.6)
The liver is the largest organ in the body and second to the
brain, performing many complex chemical and metabolic functions including the detoxification of drugs and hormones for
excretion, and the production, storage and synthesis of proteins
and blood clotting factors, filtration and storage of vitamins,
minerals and glycogen (Marieb 2006; Smith 2005b).

Interpreting liver results is complicated because some of the
enzymes involved in liver metabolism and biosynthesis are also

---

Box 9.11   Clinical context – bicarbonate

Bicarbonate is tightly regulated; when bicarbonate levels are low this is called a metabolic acidosis with associated compensatory respiratory alkalosis (hyperventilation) (Jevon & Ewens 2007). Excess bicarbonate results in a metabolic alkalosis with associated compensatory respiratory acidosis (hypoventilation).

	pH	HCO3	PaCO2 (compensatory)
Acidosis	<7.35	<22 mmol/L	<3.5 kPa
Alkalosis	>7.45	>26 mmol/L	>6.0 kPa

---

found in other organs and are not specific to the liver. There are a number of biochemical and haematological tests that provide a complete evaluation of liver function and liver disease; albumin and bilirubin primarily assess liver function; several enzymes as listed below are markers of liver disease (Beckingham 2001) and a clotting profile (PT/INR) provides information on the production of clotting factors.

Specific liver function tests
The only specific LFT is alanine aminotransferase (ALT) produced by the liver hepatocytes (Beckingham 2001).

Non-specific liver function tests
Alkaline phosphatase (ALP) is found in the liver, bone, WBCs, intestines and hepatobiliary tree (Siconolfi 1995).

Aspartate aminotransferase (AST) is found in the heart, skeletal structures, kidney and pancreas. It can be elevated after myocardial infarction, in acute pancreatitis and in liver cancer, hepatitis and cirrhosis (Siconolfi 1995) (see Box 9.12).

Plasma proteins (see Table 9.6)
Plasma proteins have many functions: coagulation, iron transport, digestive enzymes and hormonal regulatory role (e.g.

Table 9.6 Liver function and plasma protein tests

Blood (serum) test	Normal values	Clinical application	Abnormal low levels and manifestations	Abnormal high levels and manifestations	Interventions
Bilirubin (total)	3–17 μmol/L	There are two different blood tests for bilirubin: conjugated (water soluble, excreted in urine) and free or unconjugated bilirubin (insoluble, not excreted in urine). The total bilirubin combines the two		When blood bilirubin levels rise (hyperbilirubinaemia) this causes the sclera, the skin and mucous membranes to develop a yellowish tinge or jaundice Jaundice normally occurs when the bilirubin level is >40 μmol/L (Blann 2007) The urine also becomes a very dark/orange colour Elevated bilirubin levels are due to cirrhosis, hepatitis, bile duct obstruction (Marieb 2006)	Treatment will depend on the causative problem See Bloom and Webster (2006) pages 120–121. on the schematic approach to identifying further investigations, the need to exclude drug and alcohol misuse and possible differential diagnosis in relation to deranged liver function tests
Alanine aminotransferase (ALT)	5–35 IU/L >1000 IU/L sign of significant hepatitis (Beckingham 2001)	Only specific enzyme produced by the liver	Not raised in obstructive jaundice	Raised levels: hepatocellular damage (Smith 2005b) Levels are raised in liver tumour, hepatitis, cirrhosis, hepatotoxic drugs	ALP and GGT are normal in hepatitis (Beckingham 2001)

256

Blood (serum) test	Normal values	Clinical application	Abnormal low levels and manifestations	Abnormal high levels and manifestations	Interventions
Aspartate aminotransferase (AST)	6–42IU/L	Aspartate aminotransferase and ALT are called the aminotransferases	Diabetic ketoacidosis, pregnancy (Siconolfi 1995)	AST is elevated in myocardial infarction viral hepatitis, cirrhosis, obstructive jaundice and cholangitis. If AST >1000 indicates hepatitis (Smith 2005b) Non-liver causes: myocardial infarction, pancreatitis, muscle disease and muscle trauma (Siconolfi 1995)	
Alkaline phosphatase (ALP or Alk Phosp)	20–130IU/L >1000IU/L sign of cholestasis	ALP is found within the liver's Kupffer cells, it is also produced in the bone	Malnutrition, pernicious anaemia, hypothyroidism (Siconolfi 1995)	Obstructive biliary disease, primary liver cancer (hepatoma) and cirrhosis will cause ALP levels to rise Non-liver causes: rheumatoid arthritis, bone disease, hyperparathyroidism	In biliary obstruction or cholestasis ALP and GGT are raised but AST is normal (Beckingham 2001) In bone disease the calcium, phosphate and GGT should be measured If GGT normal, the problem is bone disease (Beckingham 2001)

Cont.

Table 9.6 Continued

Blood (serum) test	Normal values	Clinical application	Abnormal low levels and manifestations	Abnormal high levels and manifestations	Interventions
Gamma (γ) glutamyl transpeptidase (GGT)	Men: 10–50IU/L Women: 7–30IU/L	GGT is found in the liver, pancreas, kidney, spleen, heart and brain. It is sensitive to hepatobiliary disease and very sensitive to alcohol and phenytoin		Elevated in hepatitis, liver cancer and obstructive liver disease. Alcohol ingestion (Siconolfi 1995) Non liver causes: post myocardial infarction	GGT is important in transporting amino acids across the cell membrane
Total protein	60–80g/L	The total protein is the sum of all plasma proteins	Low protein levels are primarily due to hypoalbuminaemia		Replacement of protein can only be achieved through effective nutrition and treating the causative problem

Blood (serum) test	Normal values	Clinical application	Abnormal low levels and manifestations	Abnormal high levels and manifestations	Interventions
Albumin	35–50 g/L	Albumin is synthesised by the liver and is a measure of hepatocyte function	Reduced albumin production due to malnutrition and liver disease, redistribution of fluid into peritoneal cavity or ascites or excessive leakage, e.g. burns (Smith 2005b) Non-liver causes: sepsis, Crohn's disease, haemodilution and increased capillary permeability causing leakage into the interstitium and oedema. Other losses are from the kidney due to nephrotic syndrome	Haemoconcentration due to dehydration may provide falsely elevated albumin level	Human albumin solution (HAS) derived from pooled human serum. HAS is available in two forms 4.5% (iso-oncotic) and 20% (hyper-oncotic) solution (Park & Roe 2000). The routine replacement of albumin in severe hypoalbuminaemia remains controversial (Cochrane Injuries Group Albumin Reviewers 1998) The SAFE study (2004) compared resuscitation with saline and albumin in the intensive care unit population; the results showed that there was no difference in outcome irrespective of the baseline albumin level 20% albumin can be administered post removal of ascitic fluid to prevent cardiovascular collapse *Cont.*

Table 9.6 *Continued*

Blood (serum) test	Normal values	Clinical application	Abnormal low levels and manifestations	Abnormal high levels and manifestations	Interventions
Globulin	2.8–3.2 g/L	4 major groups of globulins: gamma, beta, alpha-2, alpha-1 globulins.	Decreased in emphysema and liver dysfunction due to α_1-antitrypsin deficiency (Beckingham 2001)	Elevated in liver disease (cirrhosis, chronic hepatitis), ulcerative colitis, chronic infections, rheumatoid arthritis and autoimmune diseases, e.g. systemic lupus	

Box 9.12 Clinical context – bilirubin formation, excretion and jaundice

Bilirubin is a by-product of red blood cell degradation, formed when the haem portion is converted via an enzymatic process into bilverdin. In turn this is then synthesised to form bilirubin. Bilirubin binds to albumin and dissociates in the liver, it is excreted in the bile and metabolised in the small intestine giving faeces its brown colour (Smith 2005b).

Bilirubin can be used to differentiate between the different causes of jaundice, which is categorised into pre-hepatic, hepatic and post-hepatic or obstructive jaundice (Beckingham & Ryder 2001).

---

insulin). They are also markers of cancer, sepsis and inflammation (Blann 2007). Gammaglobulins or immunoglobulins are produced by the immune system cells (Marieb 2006).

Albumin
Albumin accounts for over 60% of the plasma proteins (Marieb & Hoehn 2007); it has a molecular mass of 69 000 daltons (Park & Roe 2000), contributing to about 80% of the colloid osmotic pressure (Metheny 2000), thereby exerting significant effect on the capillary to keep fluid within the vascular space. Albumin is synthesised by the liver and has a long half-life of 20 days (Beckingham 2001) and a large serum pool; therefore it is a late indicator of malnutrition.

Calcium, phosphate and thyroid function (see Table 9.7)

Calcium
Calcium is found in two main forms, non-ionised and ionised. The total calcium is the sum of the ionised (50%) and non-ionised (40%) calcium. The non-ionised calcium is bound to albumin. In critical illness the ionised calcium is the most clinically important due to its role in many physiological reactions and in maintaining calcium homeostasis (see Box 9.13). Calcium has many important functions:

- transmission of nerve impulses to bring about the excitation and contractility of cardiac, skeletal and smooth muscle during the action potential

Table 9.7 Calcium, phosphate and thyroid function

Blood (serum) test	Normal values	Clinical application	Abnormal low levels and manifestations	Abnormal high levels and manifestations	Interventions
Calcium (Ca^{2+}) cation	Total corrected Ca^{2+} 2.33–2.57 mmol/L Ionised Ca 1.15–1.27 mmol/L. Available from arterial blood gas analysers	Albumin levels may affect the binding and transport of Ca^{2+} (Miller & Graham 2006) It is important to record the corrected Ca^{2+} which has been adjusted to a normal albumin (Miller & Graham 2006)	Hypocalcaemia (<2.1 mmol/L) may be due to alkalosis; this increases calcium and albumin binding, chronic renal failure, pancreatitis, sepsis, toxic shock syndrome, low magnesium and phosphate levels, primary hypothyroidism (Metheny 2000) and poor oral intake of calcium and vitamin D (Blann 2007) In hypoalbuminaemia the calcium level may not be low but may appear so due to the low albumin level (Miller & Graham 2006) Cardiac clinical signs of hypocalcaemia include bradycardia, prolonged QT interval, T wave inversion, cardiac arrest (Resuscitation Council 2010). Congestive cardiac failure (CCF) due to impaired myocardial function The most common manifestation is tetany characterised by a varying range in severity of neurological symptoms; muscle contractions and spasm seizures and hallucinations (Miller & Graham 2006)	The main cause of hypercalcaemia (>2.6 mmol/L) is hyperparathyroidism due to increased parathyroid hormone (PTH) levels often due to tumour (mainly bony metastases) and other malignancies, sarcoidosis and myeloma Thiazides and lithium decrease the excretion of calcium Overuse of vitamin and calcium supplements and post renal transplantation can all elevate calcium levels Clinical signs of hypercalcaemia: patients are often asymptomatic but hypercalcaemia can cause vomiting, abdominal pain, pancreatitis, and at higher levels myocardial depression can occur (Miller & Graham 2006), leading to arrhythmias and cardiac arrest (Resuscitation Council 2010) Confusion, weakness and hypotension are other manifestations (Resuscitation Council 2010)	The treatment for hypercalcaemia depends on the causative problem In severe hypocalcaemia or during cardiac arrest calcium chloride 10% 10–40 mL IV is administered. (Resuscitation Council 2010) Magnesium sulphate should also be used to optimise magnesium levels prior to replenishing calcium Other blood tests that should also be carried out include PTH, Mg, K and creatinine levels (Miller & Graham 2006)

Cont.

Phosphate (PO_4^{2-}) anion	0.81– 1.45 mmol/L	Haemolysis or damage to the RBCs during blood sampling will cause release of PO_4^{2-} into the serum, invalidating the results	Severe hypophosphataemia (<0.4 mmol/L) can be caused by respiratory alkalosis, alcohol withdrawal, acute liver failure An increased phosphorus level should be analysed in the context of the calcium level as the two have an inverse relationship (Metheny 2000) Chronic renal failure
Parathyroid hormone (PTH)	10–65 ng/L		Low PTH levels can lead to tetany and death High PTH levels are rare and due mainly to parathyroid tumour
Thyroid stimulating hormone (TSH)	0.4– 4.5 mU/L	Concentrations tend to be higher at night and there is variation between laboratories (BTA 2006)	Hyperthyroidism or thyrotoxicosis is associated in the elderly with depression, weight loss and exacerbation of existing cardiovascular problems, e.g. atrial fibrillation (British Thyroid Association 2006) Other causes include Graves' disease characterised by goitre (enlarged thyroid gland) and protuberance of the eyes or exophthalmia. TSH levels are low but T3 and T4 are elevated (see T4 hypersecretion effects)	Elevated levels of TSH (>10 mU/L) are diagnostic of primary hypothyroidism (Vaidya & Pearce 2008). There are many clinical signs associated with hypothyroidism including exhaustion, weight gain, depression, bradycardia and dry, thin pale skin (Vaidya & Pearce 2008) Causes of hypothyroidism are varied including autoimmune diseases, iodine deficiency, drugs such as amiodarone, lithium, rifampicin, pituitary and hypothalamus disorders, thyroiditis (Vaidya & Pearce 2008)

Table 9.7 *Continued*

Blood (serum) test	Normal values	Clinical application	Abnormal low levels and manifestations	Abnormal high levels and manifestations	Interventions
Free T4 (thyroxine)	9.0–25 pmol/L		Hyposecretion causes decreased body temperature and glucose metabolism, bradycardia and hypotension, sluggish muscle actions, decreased gut motility	Hypersecretion causes increased temperature and basal metabolic rate, irritability, tachycardia; elevated blood pressure, diarrhoea and anorexia due to hyperstimulation of the gastrointestinal tract, weight loss (Wallace 2005)	

Box 9.13   Clinical context – calcium levels

Ninety-nine per cent of calcium is found in bones (Blann 2007). The remaining 1% is found within the ICF (9/10) and ECF (1/10). Ten per cent of calcium is chelated (bound) to bicarbonate, lactate, phosphate citrate and ketones (Venkatesh 2003), which can affect calcium levels in lactic acidosis. Metabolic alkalosis can lower calcium levels due to increased binding to albumin.

- heart rate control, preservation of the automaticity properties of cardiac cells and prevention of arrhythmias (Metheny 2000)
- essential component for many of the enzyme-dependent reactions required for the activation of the coagulation pathways (Breen 2004).

Phosphate

Phosphate is an intracellular ion present as creatine phosphate or adenosine triphosphate (e.g. ATP). ATP is formed of high-energy phosphate bonds which when the phosphate group is cleaved release their energy to enable cellular processes to occur (Smith 2005a). Phosphate is also present in RBC in the compound 2,3-diphosphoglycerate. Eighty-five percent of phosphate is found in the bone, which acts as a reservoir (Blann 2007).

Thyroid function

Thyroid hormone is composed of two hormones, thyroxine (T4) and triiodothyronine (T3). The release of both hormones is triggered by feedback mechanisms. Both hormones have a multitude of physiological effects.

Parathyroid hormone (PTH) released by the parathyroid glands regulates calcium balance; reduced circulating calcium ion levels trigger the release of PTH, which stimulates the skeleton to release calcium and phosphates into the blood (Metheny 2000). PTH stimulates the kidney to promote vitamin D activation and the intestine to increase the absorption of calcium from food (Wallace 2005). Due to the inverse relationship between calcium and phosphate if the concentration of one rises, the other is reduced and vice versa (Metheny 2000).

Cardiac markers: monitoring cardiac function and disease (see Table 9.8)

The assessment of cardiac function and arterial circulation for atherosclerosis and diabetes is vital in reducing the burden of ischemic heart disease, stroke and obesity throughout the United Kingdom (DH 2000). Damaged cardiac myocytes release intracellular proteins into the bloodstream; newer blood tests such as troponin (proteins) are much more specific compared to traditional enzymes (Jowett & Thompson 2003). Table 9.8 summarises the blood tests performed to detect and monitor for myocardial injury, hyperlipidaemia and diabetes.

Acute phase proteins (see Table 9.9)

Acute phase proteins are useful in monitoring the body's response to interventions and the course of inflammatory and infectious process (Marieb & Hoehn 2007).

Additional biochemistry tests

Lactate (see Table 9.10)

Lactate is produced by the skin, erythrocytes and skeletal muscle; lactate concentration within the cell is regulated by the pyruvate cycle (Marieb & Hoehn 2007). The kidneys and liver are the main organs of lactate metabolism and excretion (Marieb & Hoehn 2007) (see Box 9.14).

Magnesium

Magnesium is mainly found in the skeleton with about one third in the intracellular fluid (Metheny 2000). Magnesium is involved in many biochemical functions; it is important in reducing myocardial irritability and arrhythmias, in enzymatic reactions, and in neuromuscular transmission. As with potassium, magnesium is excreted via the kidney.

Magnesium has many properties, often being called 'magic magnesium'. It is recommended by the British Thoracic Society (BTS) in the management guideline for acute asthma (2008). In

Table 9.8 Blood tests for cardiac function, hyperlipidaemia and diabetes mellitus

Blood (serum) test	Normal values	Clinical application	Abnormal low levels and manifestations	Abnormal high levels and manifestations	Interventions
Creatine kinase (CK)	Male 15–160 IU/L Female 15–130 IU/L	Found in skeletal, cardiac muscle and the brain		Released post myocardial infarction or myocardial injury and skeletal muscle injuries, e.g. rhabdomyolysis (Russell 2000)	
CK-MB ratio	<25 IU/L	CK-MB is specific for myocardial tissue		Elevated post myocardial infarction, CK-MB rises within 4–8 hours, peaks at 12–24 hours, and disappears by 72 hours (Jowett & Thompson 2003). Angina, cardiac contusions also increase CK-MB (Olbrych 1993)	

Cont.

Table 9.8 *Continued*

Blood (serum) test	Normal values	Clinical application	Abnormal low levels and manifestations	Abnormal high levels and manifestations	Interventions
Troponin	Troponin T = 0.01–0.1 μg/L (upper limit of normal) Troponin I = 0.1–2 μg/L; detection around 0.007 μg/L	There are 3 cardiac troponins, T, I and C. Troponins are proteins bound to skeletal and cardiac myocytes (Jowett & Thompson 2003)		Troponin T and I are sensitive markers for myocardial injury. Within 3–4 hours of myocardial injury troponin T and I are released peaking at 12–24 hours. They remain raised for 4–10 days (Ammann *et al.* 2004) Troponins are also raised in critically ill patients, high dose chemotherapy, pulmonary embolism, renal failure, sepsis and septic shock, stroke, subarachnoid haemorrhage (Ammann *et al.* 2004)	Interpretation of elevated troponins must be considered along with the history and clinical examination

Lactate dehydrogenase (LDH)	70–250 IU/L	Enzyme found in most body tissues; released when there is cell damage	If liver enzymes are deranged and the LDH is elevated the primary cause might be the liver. Other causes include kidney disease, stroke, pancreatitis, tumours, haemolytic anaemia and muscular dystrophy Strenuous exercise can cause a temporary rise (Lab Tests Online 2007)	Troponin testing has largely replaced the use of LDH as a marker of cardiac disease
Total cholesterol	2.5– 5.0 mmol/L	Cholesterol and triglycerides are the main lipids monitored	Malabsorption syndrome, sepsis, anaemia liver disease (Siconolfi 1995)	Increased levels are often genetically linked, and associated with biliary cirrhosis, hyperlipidaemia, diabetes, hypertension, arterial disease or atherosclerosis, myocardial infarction and coronary artery heart disease (Jowett & Thompson 2003)

Cont.

Table 9.8 Continued

Blood (serum) test	Normal values	Clinical application	Abnormal low levels and manifestations	Abnormal high levels and manifestations	Interventions
Triglycerides	<2.3 mmol/L	Along with cholesterol helps to determine the risk for developing atherosclerosis and heart disease		Hypertriglyceridaemia can cause pancreatitis (Jowett & Thompson 2003)	

Fasting blood glucose	<6.1 mmol/L	Fasting blood glucose is performed to determine the presence of diabetes A grey coloured bottle top is used; glucose is not performed on clotted blood	Hypoglycaemia is defined as blood glucose <2.8 mmol/L. Clinical signs include changes in behaviour and confusion. If left it leads to coma and death Causes of hypoglycaemia: hepatic failure causes depleted glycogen stores and increased insulin levels (Hawker 2003). Addison's disease, overdose of insulin, myxoedema, coma and rebound hypoglycaemia if total parenteral nutrition (TPN) is stopped suddenly	Hyperglycaemia >10 mmol/L may be a sign of undiagnosed diabetes mellitus or a marker of insulin resistance associated with sepsis or endothelial dysfunction	Diabetes is diagnosed on one the following blood tests and the presence of any symptoms, e.g. polyuria: Fasting glucose >7.0 mmol/L Random glucose >11.1 mmol/L or formal oral glucose–tolerance test (OGTT) (Jowett & Thompson 2003)

Table 9.9 Acute phase proteins

Blood (serum) test	Normal values	Clinical application	Abnormal low levels and manifestations	Abnormal high levels and manifestations
C-reactive protein	<5 mg/L Mean 2.4 mg/L	Acute phase marker for tissue injury, infection, inflammation and malignancy. It is useful in monitoring the body's response to interventions and course of the inflammatory /infectious process (Marieb & Hoehn 2007)		The CRP can be raised even when the WBC is normal or low

Table 9.10 Additional blood tests

Blood (serum) test	Normal values	Clinical application	Abnormal low levels and manifestations	Abnormal high levels and manifestations	Interventions
Lactate	0/6–1.7 mmol/L Venous blood	Venous samples might yield slightly higher values than arterial sampling. Hand clenching can raise the lactate level (Metheny 2000). Arterial blood gas sampling is also problematic due to the multiple causes of metabolic acidosis (Bakker 1996)		Elevated lactate levels are seen in severe sepsis and haemorrhagic shock leading to oxygen debt (Bakker 1996)	

Cont.

Table 9.10 *Continued*

Blood (serum) test	Normal values	Clinical application	Abnormal low levels and manifestations	Abnormal high levels and manifestations	Interventions
Magnesium (Mg^{2+}) Second main intracellular cation to potassium	0.75–1.05 mmol/L	Serum magnesium is relatively low; therefore actual cellular magnesium may be much lower than the measured serum level. Haemolysis or damage to the RBC during blood sampling will cause release of Mg^{2+} into the serum, invalidating the results	Hypomagnesaemia can be caused by a variety of clinical problems, starvation, TPN, chronic alcoholism and increased losses from the kidney. Magnesium is lost from the gut and is redistributed in pancreatitis and burns (Metheny 2000) Clinical signs include muscle weakness and cramps, cardiac arrhythmias, coronary artery spasm, hypokalaemia and insomnia	Hypermagnesaemia can cause cardiac arrest due to increased PR and QT intervals at levels exceeding 15–20 mmol/L. Magnesium toxicity can be caused by renal failure (most common cause), over-administration of magnesium and magnesium containing antacids. Clinical signs vary according to the degree of toxicity. At 3–5 mmol/L symptoms include nausea and vomiting, flushing, vasodilatation and hypotension. At 4–7 mmol/L, muscle weakness and loss of deep tendon reflexes occurs, and at 10–15 mmol/L respiratory paralysis occurs (Metheny 2000)	Replenishing magnesium and maintaining therapeutic levels is vitally important for reducing the incidence of life-threatening arrhythmias and cardiac arrest and maintaining transcellular function
Amylase	Male 60–180 IU/L Female 95–290 IU/L	Diagnostic for pancreatitis. Amylase is an enzyme which digests starch		Released following pancreatitis, mumps and parotid gland swelling. Amylase levels rise 2–12 hours after the onset of symptoms. Peaks at 12–72 hours. It may rise to 5–10 times the normal level and returns to normal level within a week	

Box 9.14 Clinical context – lactate levels

Monitoring of lactate levels may reveal tissue hypoxia due to low cardiac output and hypoperfusion resulting in a sluggish circulation and poor tissue perfusion. Normal cellular metabolism requires oxygen for aerobic respiration; changes in oxygen delivery and cellular consumption in anaerobic situations (without oxygen) increase lactate production. Lactic acid is a weak acid and is said to be present when the blood lactate level exceeds 4–5 mmol/L (Metheny 2000).

---

pre-eclampsia the mechanism of action is not fully understood, but it is thought to act as a smooth muscle relaxant bringing about vasodilation as well as anticonvulsant properties (Duley & Henderson-Smart 2003).

Amylase
The amylase test is primarily performed when pancreatitis is suspected. Amylase is a digestive enzyme normally released by the salivary glands and pancreas. Pancreatitis can be either an acute or chronic inflammatory process, whereby the release of amylase and other tissue necrosing factors induces autodigestion of pancreatic tissue, leading to swelling, haemorrhage and worsening pancreatic failure. Elevated amylase levels are not prognostic for outcome.

CONCLUSION
Understanding the meaning of blood results, which blood tests to request for different disease processes and then acting on those results is an important role for nurses. This chapter has outlined some of the core knowledge required in order to facilitate application to clinical context of a complex subject.

REFERENCES
Ammann, P., Pfisterer, M., Fehr, T. & Rickli, H. (2004) Raised cardiac troponins. *BMJ*, **328**, 1028–1029.

Anastasiou, C.A., Kavouras, S.A., Arnaoutis, G., Gioxari Am Kollia, M., Botoula, E. & Sidossis, L.S. (2009) Sodium replacement and plasma sodium droop during exercise in the heat when fluid intake matches fluid loss. *Journal of Athletic Training*, **44**(2), 117–123.

Andrews, N.C. (1999) Disorders of iron metabolism. *New England Journal of Medicine*, **341**(26), 1986–1995.

Arieff, A.I. (1993) Management of hyponatraemia. *BMJ*, **307**(6899), 305–308.

Bakker, J. (1996) Monitoring of blood lactate levels: a guide to therapy to improve tissue oxygenation. *International Journal of Intensive Care*, **3**(1), 29–39.

Bannister, A.B., Begg, N.T. & Gillespie, S.H. (1996) *Infectious Disease*. Blackwell Science, Oxford.

Beckingham, I.J. (2001) *ABC of Liver, Pancreas and Gall Bladder*. BMJ Books, London.

Beckingham, I.J. & Ryder, S.D. (2001) Investigation of liver and biliary disease. In: *ABC of Liver, Pancreas and Gall Bladder* (ed. I. Beckingham), pp 1–4. BMJ Books, London.

Blann, A. (2007) *Routine Blood Results Explained*, 2nd edn. M&K Update Ltd, Cumbria.

Bloom, S. & Webster, G. (2006) *Oxford Handbook of Gastroenterology and Hepatology*. Oxford University Press, Oxford.

Bratt-Wyton, R. (1998) Interpretation of routine blood results. *Nursing Standard*, **13**(12), 42–48.

Breen, P. (2004) Basics of coagulation pathways. *International Journal of Anaesthesiology Clinics*, **42**(3), 1–9.

British Thoracic Society Scottish Intercollegiate Guidelines Network (2008) British Guideline on the Management of Asthma. *Thorax*, **63**(Suppl. 4).

British Thyroid Association (2006) UK guidelines for the use of thyroid function tests. TFT guideline final version (2006) at http://www.british-thyroid-association.org/info-forpatients/ Docs/TFT_guideline_final_version_July_2006.pdf (accessed 30 November 2009).

Chapman, J.F., Elliott, C., Knowles, S.M., Milkins, C.E., Poole, G.D.; Working Party of the British Committee for Standards in Haematology Blood Transfusion Task Force (2004) Guidelines for compatibility procedures in blood transfusion laboratories. *Transfusion Medicine*, **14**, 59–73.

Coats, T.J., Brazil, E. & Heron, M. (2006) The effects of commonly used resuscitation fluids on whole blood coagulation. *Emergency Medicine Journal*, **23**, 546–549.

Cochrane Injuries Group Albumin Reviewers (1998) Human albumin administration in critically ill patients: systematic review of randomised controlled trials. *BMJ*, **317**, 235–240.

Contreras, M. & Mijovic, A. (2009) Compatibility testing before transfusion; blood ordering and administration. In: *ABC of Transfusion* (ed. M. Contreras), 4edn, Chap. 3. Wiley-Blackwells, Oxford.

Criddle, L. (2006) A pinch of salt: dealing with hyponatremic emergencies. *American Journal of Nursing*, **106**(10), 72CC–72EE.

Department of Health (2000) *Coronary Heart Disease National Service Framework*. The Stationery Office, London.

Department of Health (2006) *Immunisations Against Infectious Diseases* (eds D. Salisbury, M. Ramsay & K. Noakes), 3rd edn. The Stationery Office, London.

Duley, L. & Henderson-Smart, D.J. (2003) Magnesium sulphate versus diazepam for eclampsia. *Cochrane Database of Systematic Reviews*, Issue 4.

Edwards, S. (2001) Regulation of water, sodium and potassium: implications for practice. *Nursing Standard*, **15**(22), 36–45.

Elias, E. & Hawkins, C. (1985) *Lecture Notes on Gastroenterology*. Blackwell Scientific Publications, Oxford.

Fox, M.A. & Fox, J.A. (2007) Acute symptomatic hyponatraemia. *Acute Medicine*, **6**, issue 3.

Hambley, H. (1995) Coagulation (II). Clinical problems in coagulation disorders. *Care of the Critically Ill*, **11**(5), 203–205.

Handy, J.M. & Soni, N. (2008) Physiological effects of hyperchloraemia and acidosis. *British Journal of Anaesthesia*, **101**(2), 141–150.

Hawker, F. (2003) Hepatic failure. In: *Oh's Intensive Care Manual* (eds A.D. Bersten & N. Soni), 5th edn. Butterworth Heinemann, Edinburgh.

Holm, E.A., Bie, P., Ottesen, M., Ødum, L. & Jespersen, B. (2009) Diagnosis of the syndrome of inappropriate secretion of antidiuretic hormone. *Southern Medical Journal*, **102**(4), 380–384.

Higgins, C. (1997) Blood coagulation: what screening tests can show. *Nursing Times*, **93**(25), 44–46.

Holt, A. (2008) Management of cardiac arrhythmias. In: *Oh's Intensive Care Manual* (eds A.D. Bersten & N. Soni), 5th edn, pp. 189–244. Butterworth Heinemann, Edinburgh.

Holum, J.R. (1998) *Fundamentals of General, Organic and Biological Chemistry*, 6th edn. John Wiley and Sons Inc., New York.

Humphreys, M. (2007) Potassium disturbances and associated electrocardiogram changes. *Emergency Nurse*, **15**(5), 28–34.

Isbister, J.P. (2003) Haemostatic failure. In: *Oh's Intensive Care Manual* (eds A.D. Bersten & N. Soni), 5th edn. Butterworth Heinemann, Edinburgh.

ISD – Information Services Division (2008) The cost book available at: http://www.isdscotland.org/isd/costs-book-detailedtables.jsp?pContentID=3584&p_applic=CCC&p_service=Content.show& (accessed 9 November 2009).

Jamieson, M.J. (1985) Hyponatraemia. *BMJ*, **290**(6483), 1723–1728.

Jevon, P. & Ewens, B. (2007) *Monitoring the Critically Ill Patient. Essential Clinical Skills for Nurses*, 2nd edn. Blackwells, Oxford.

Jowett, N.I. & Thompson, D.R. (2003) *Comprehensive Coronary Care*, 3rd edn. Baillière Tindall, London.

Knoll, M.H. & Elin, R.J. (1994) Interference with clinical laboratory analyses. *Clinical Chemistry*, **40**(11), 1996–2005.

Lab Tests Online (2007) http://www.labtestsonline.org (accessed 2 September 2009).

Levi, M. & Cate, H.T. (1999) Disseminated intravascular coagulation. *New England Journal of Medicine*, **341**, 586–592.

Lippi, G., Montagnana, M., Salvagno, G.L. & Guidi, G.C. (2006) Interference of blood cell lysis on routine coagulation testing. *Archives of Pathology and Laboratory Medicine*, **130**(44), 181–184.

Mahoney, B., Smith, W., Lo, D., Tsoi, K., Tonelli, M. & Clase, C. (2005) Emergency interventions for hyperkalaemia. *Cochrane Database of Systematic Reviews*, CD003235.

Marieb, E. (2006) *Essentials of Human Anatomy and Physiology*, 8th edn. Pearson Benjamin Cummings, USA.

Marieb, E. & Hoehn, K. (2007) *Human Anatomy and Physiology*, 7th edn. Pearson International, USA.

Martin, L. (1999) *All You Really Need To Know To Interpret Arterial Blood Gases*, 2nd edn. Lippincott Williams & Wilkins, Baltimore.

McCall, R. & Tankersley, C.M. (2008) *Phlebotomy Essentials Workbook*, 4th edn. Lippincott Williams & Wilkins, Philadelphia.

McClelland, D.B.L. (2007) *Handbook of Transfusion Medicine*, 4th edn. UK Blood Services; The Stationery Office, London.

McLaren, S.M. (2005) Renal function. In: *Physiology for Nursing Practice* (eds S. Montague *et al.*), 3rd edn. pp. 595–632. Baillière Tindall, UK.

Metheny, N.M. (2000) *Fluid and Electrolyte Balance: Nursing Considerations*, 4th edn. Lippincott Williams & Wilkins, Philadelphia.

Miller, W. & Graham, M.G. (2006) Life-threatening electrolyte abnormalities Patient Care on line http://www.modernmedicine. com/modernmedicine/Metabolic+disorders/Life-threatening-electrolyte-abnormalities/ArticleStandard/Article/detail/391516 (accessed 30 November 2009).

Minors, D.S. (2001) Blood cells, haemoglobin, haemostasis and coagulation. *Anaesthesia and Intensive Care Medicine*, **2**(4), 149–154.

Montague, S.E. (2005) The blood. In: *Physiology for Nursing Practice* (eds S. Montague *et al.*), 3rd edn, pp. 335–381. Baillière Tindall, UK.

NBS – National Blood Service (2008) *Transfusion Matters: The Journey of a Bag of Blood from Hospital Laboratory to Patient*, 5th edn. (Summer/Autumn) p 1–4. AT: http://www.bbts.org.uk/PDFs/education/12%2008%2008%20-%2020206%20Transfusion%20Matters-4pp.pdf (accessed 30 November 2009).

NICE – National Institute for Health and Clinical Excellence (2008) Identifying and treating long-term kidney problems (chronic kidney disease). At: http://nice.org.uk/CG73 (accessed 26 September 2010).

Park, R. & Roe, G. (2000) *Fluid Balance and Volume Resuscitation for Beginners*. Greenwich Medical Media, London.

Patel, M. (2007) Asymptomatic hyponatraemia on the acute medical unit. *Acute Medicine*, **6**(3), 108–113.

Olbrych, D.D. (1993) Interpreting C.P.K. *Nursing*, **23**(1), 48–49.

Park, R. & Roe, G. (2000) *Fluid Balance and Volume Resuscitation for Beginners*. Cambridge University Press, Cambridge.

Parker, L.J. (2002) Infection and disease. In: *Watson's Clinical Nursing and Related Sciences* (ed. M. Walsh), 6th edn, pp. 125–149. Baillière Tindall, London.

Perez, A. (1995) Electrolytes: restoring the balance. Hyperkalaemia. *RN*, **58**(11), 32–37.

Reid, J.L., Rubin, P.C. & Walters, M.R. (2006) *Clinical Pharmacology and Therapeutics*. Blackwell Publishing. Oxford.

Rempher, K.J. & Little, J. (2004) Assessment of red blood cell and coagulation laboratory data. *AACN Clinical Issues*, **15**(4), 622–637.

Resuscitation Council (UK) (2010) *Advanced Life Support*, 6th edn. London.

Reynolds, R.M., Padfield, P.L. & Seckl, J.R. (2006) Disorders of sodium balance. *BMJ*, **332**(7543), 702–705.

Rosenson, R.S., Staffileno, B.A. & Tangney, C.C. (1998) Effects of tourniquet technique, order of draw, and sample storage on plasma fibrinogen. *Clinical Chemistry*, **44**, 688–690.

Russell, T.A. (2000) Acute renal failure related to rhabdomyolysis: pathophysiology, diagnosis and collaborative management. *Nephrology Nursing Journal*, **27**(6), 567–575.

Siconolfi, L.A. (1995) Clarifying the complexity of liver function tests. *Nursing*, **25**(5), 39–45.

Smith, G.D (2005a) The acquisition of nutrients. In: *Physiology for Nursing Practice* (eds S. Montague *et al.*), pp. 467–514, 3rd edn. Baillière Tindall, UK.

Smith, G.D (2005b) The liver. In: *Physiology for Nursing Practice* (eds S. Montague *et al.*), 3rd edn. Baillière Tindall, UK.

Stark, J.L. (1994) Interpreting B.U.N./creatinine levels. It's not as simple as you think. *Nursing*, **24**(9), 58–61.

Sterns, R.H. & Silver, S.M. (2003) Salt and water: read the package insert. *Q J Med*, **96**, 549–552.

SAFE Study Investigators (2004) A comparison of albumin and saline for fluid resuscitation in the intensive care unit. *New England Journal of Medicine*, **350**(22), 2247–2256.

Tillyard, A., Keays, R. & Soni, N. (2005) The diagnosis of acute renal failure in intensive care: mongrel or pedigree. *Anaesthesia*, **60**, 903–914.

Traynor, J., Mactier, R., Geddes, C.C. & Fox, J.G. (2006) How to measure renal function in clinical practice. *BMJ*, **333**(7571), 733–737.

Vaidya, B. & Pearce, S.H.S. (2008) Management of hypothyroidism in adults. *BMJ*, **337**, a801.

Vedig, A.Ee (2003) Diabetes insipidus. In: *Oh's Intensive Care Manual* (eds A.D. Bersten & N. Soni), 5th edn. Butterworth Heinemann, Edinburgh.

Venkatesh, B (2003) Acute calcium disorders. In: *Oh's Intensive Care Manual* (eds A.D. Bersten & N. Soni), 5th edn. Butterworth Heinemann, Edinburgh.

Wallace, W.F.M. (2005) Endocrine function. In: *Physiology for Nursing Practice* (eds S. Montague *et al.*), 3rd edn, pp. 207–250. Baillière Tindall, UK.

Watson, R. (2000) Altered presentation in old age. *Elderly Care*, **12**(3), 19–21.

Woodrow, P. (2003a) Assessing blood results in older people: haematology and liver function tests. *Nursing Older People*, **15**(3), 29–31.

Woodrow, P. (2003b) Assessing blood results in older people: cardiac enzymes and biochemistry. *Nursing Older People*, **15**(4), 31–33.

Worthley, L.I.G. (2003) Fluid and electrolyte therapy. In: *Oh's Intensive Care Manual* (eds A.D. Bersten & N. Soni), 5th edn. Butterworth Heinemann, Edinburgh.

Patient's Perspective

10

Lisa Dougherty

LEARNING OUTCOMES

The practitioner will be able to:
- ❏ Have an understanding of the causes of blood and injection phobias.
- ❏ Identify factors that influence pain and anxiety.
- ❏ Discuss the techniques that can reduce pain including pharmacological and non-pharmacological methods.

INTRODUCTION

> If you get a first good injection then it will never be worse than that.
>
> (Dougherty 1994)

The influence of a bad experience can be overwhelming for a patient and any practitioner performing venepuncture or cannulation must never underestimate either the impact for the patient of undergoing the procedure or how they may view either procedure in the future. Anxiety can be caused by previous bad experience, a degree of needle phobia or dislike of needle procedures (Lavery & Ingram 2005).

BLOOD AND INJECTION PHOBIA

Definition

Phobias are a special form of fear, disproportionate to the situation in which it occurs (Koppel 1999). Blood and injection phobias are specific phobias. The definition of a specific phobia

Venepuncture and Cannulation, first edition. Edited by Sarah Phillips, Mary Collins and Lisa Dougherty. Published 2011 by Blackwell Publishing Ltd. © 2011 Blackwell Publishing Ltd.

is 'a clinically significant anxiety provoked by exposure to a specified feared object or situation often leading to avoidance behaviour' (APA 2000).

Blood needle phobias are common and potentially life-threatening. It is estimated that these phobias may occur up to 3.5–4% of the time, in varying degrees of severity, in a person's lifetime (Koppel 1999; Patel *et al.* 2005). The degree of anxiety depends on the perceived risk or proximity of blood and needles therefore needles seen on the TV are less likely to produce the same level of anxiety as those seen in real life (Stark & Brener 2000).

Phobias have a tendency to develop in childhood and then appear to be exaggerated beyond the normal childhood developmental fear. No absolute, definitive singular causal model adequately explains why some people develop phobias and others do not. It is considered that developmental learning has a role to play through direct conditioning, vicarious conditioning (observing another person's fear) or by the transmission of information or instruction (Rogers & Gournay 2001).

Features

- Marked and persistent fear that is excessive or unreasonable, cued by the presence of or anticipation of a specific object or situation (e.g. seeing blood or receiving injections).
- Exposure to triggers causes an immediate and intense anxiety response or panic.
- Individual has insight that his/her fear is excessive.
- Trigger situations are either avoided or tolerated but with intense distress and anxiety.
- Disorder has significant effects on the person's ability to maintain everyday activities.
- Fear is not better explained by another disorder (Stark & Brener 2000; Rogers & Gournay 2001).

Manifestations of a phobia

- **Behavioural:** avoidance triggers for their anxiety.
- **Cognitive:** there are many different manifestations; fear of fainting is one associated with injection, making patients more anxious.

- **Physiological:** panic, palpitations, breathlessness. The physiology of blood injection injury phobia manifests initially as tachycardia, followed by vasovagal bradycardia, drop in blood pressure, ending in fainting – approximately 75% of individuals report fainting (Stark & Brener 2000; Rogers & Gournay 2001).

Management of phobias

1. **Referral:** Referral to nurse therapists and self-help groups (e.g. Triumph over Phobias – TOPS) can be useful.
2. **Systemic desensitisation/exposure therapy:** This requires a baseline measurement of anxiety and then gradual and repeated exposure to the feared stimulus, to reduce associated anxiety and distress. This may be difficult as patients with blood needle phobia are more prone to fainting during this therapy (Koppel 1999; Rogers & Gournay 2001).
3. **Cognitive behavioural therapy:** A range of specific techniques that include identification of negative thoughts and appraisals, role plays and behavioural experiments.
4. **Medication:**
   - Selective serotonin reuptake inhibitors (SSRIs) have some potential benefits.
   - Low-dose propranolol benefits a third of cases.
   - Routine use of benzodiazepines is rare due to risk of dependency (Rogers & Gournay 2001).

FACTORS THAT CAN INFLUENCE PAIN AND ANXIETY

Age

Age appears to play a role in the amount of pain and distress associated with needles. Agras *et al.* (1969) showed that the incidence of injection fear in the general population rises sharply from 0 to 15 years and then there is a steep decline ending at 30 years of age, suggesting that the fear is short-lived. However, both Wilson-Barnett (1976) and Coates *et al.* (1983) found that hospitalised patients under 40 years of age responded more negatively to injections than did those aged 40 and over. Age has also been correlated to the level of distress associated with routine venepuncture (Bennett-Humphrey & Boon 1992).

Gender

A study of cancer patients by Coates *et al.* (1983) to discover what caused the most distress during chemotherapy revealed that 'having a needle' was ranked as the sixth most distressing. This study was repeated in 1993 (Griffin *et al.* 1996) when fear of a needle was ranked in the top five most severe side effects by more women than men and this finding was statistically significant.

The literature has explored the influence of gender on pain and anxiety. Van den Berg & Abeysekera (1993) found that female patients tended to have greater pain scores and more responses during the cannulation procedure, suggesting that female patients may need more care and attention than male patients during the procedure. Miaskowski (1997) found that studies indicate that women exhibit lower pain thresholds than men and also exhibit less tolerance to noxious stimuli than men. This is supported by Berkley (1997) but both report that studies were small, exist only for certain forms of stimulus and are affected by situational variables such as disease. Results may also be explained by hormonal status as well as being influenced by the gender of the experimenter.

However, it must be remembered that men tend to have been socialised to appear brave and not express pain (Levine & De Simone 1991). Men have reported less pain in front of female than male experimenters although this did not influence responses in females. In contrast at least two studies showed that gender differences in pain sensitivity were not affected by the gender of the experimenter (Otto & Dougher 1985; Feine *et al.*, 1991). Berkley (1997) also reported on a study where views relating to anticipation of pain of an impending venepuncture differed between male and female children but there were no differences in rates of the pain actually produced. Kelley *et al.* (1997) compared pain and distress in women undergoing urethral catheterisation with women undergoing peripheral venous cannulation. Distress levels were the same for both procedures but cannulation caused more pain. What appears to be key is that attitudes towards pain can affect coping mechanisms and therefore response to treatment.

Aspects that can improve the experience

Many patients will be apprehensive and this anxiety may cause vasoconstriction – making venepuncture or cannulation more difficult for patient and practitioner and more painful for the patient. How the nurse approaches the patient, her manner and attitude, may give a direct bearing on the patient's response to the procedure (Weinstein 2007). Although routine to the nurse it may be a new and frightening experience for the patient unfamiliar with the procedure (Weinstein 2007). Patients should be approached in a calm and reassuring manner and encouraged to ask questions and share prior experience of venepuncture or cannulation, good or bad, as this can affect the patient's acceptance of treatment and reduce anxiety (Lavery & Ingram 2005). If the patient's history includes complications associated with either procedure, venepuncture or cannulation may be very difficult (Weinstein 2007). However, when the procedures are performed by an experienced practitioner and it is a positive experience for the patient, he or she may feel more comfortable and relaxed. Provision of clear and comprehensive information on the procedure should reduce the patient's anxiety and pain (Lücker & Stahlheber-Dilg 2003; Weinstein 2007; Dougherty 2008).

TECHNIQUES TO REDUCE ANXIETY AND PAIN

Ernst & Ernst (2001) listed four secrets to a painless venepuncture:

- vein choice
- needle size/type
- good anchoring
- allowing the skin to dry following disinfection, to prevent a burning sensation of alcohol when the skin is punctured.

Vein choice

Many patients find that use of the antecubital vein brings less discomfort for venepuncture than use of the cephalic and basilic veins. This may be due to the close proximity of the median antebrachial cutaneous nerve to the basilic vein (Ernst & Ernst

2001). Hefler *et al.* (2004) found that patients felt the least discomfort when the antecubital fossa was used followed by the forearm, the back of the hand and lastly the radial aspect of the wrist. However, it is more likely that the pain during venepuncture or cannulation originates from nerve fibres in the skin rather than the blood vessel (Scales 2008) as veins have no innervation. Nerve fibres under the skin react to the temperature, pressure, touch and pain. The number of nerve fibres varies in different areas of the body. Some areas are highly sensitive, and insertion of a needle results in a great deal of pain such as the inner aspect of the wrist, whilst others are only mildly sensitive (Weinstein 2007). Palpating and cleaning the skin triggers multiple sensory pathways to the brain. These in turn may trigger memories of previous experiences resulting in pain being anticipated even before cannulation (Scales 2005).

Needle size and type
Lücker & Stahlheber (2003) compared types of cannulae to see if this influenced pain. Whilst they found differences in pain, ease of insertion and flashback, they concluded that a clinician's choice of cannula is made after considering a variety of factors and the clinician's perception of ease in using the device, and therefore ease of insertion, may result in a reduction in pain experienced by the patient. A study by Van den Berg & Abeysekera (1993) investigating venous cannulation in a large sample of patients (1422) considered a range of influencing factors during the insertion of a cannula. These included arm used, vein site, cannula size and pain on cannulation. Pain was assessed by a verbal analogue scale and observation of patients' responses. Use of the cephalic vein and a larger gauge (16G) cannula produced more responses, but reported pain was reduced when lidocaine was used. Cannula design has also been implicated in the degree of reported pain, with thin-walled cannulae appearing to cause less pain than thick-walled cannulae (Ahrens *et al.* 1991). Ahrens *et al.* (1991) also found that patients feel more pain with each subsequent attempt at cannulation. It could therefore be suggested that better success rates will be achieved by more experienced staff and this in turn will reduce pain and anxiety.

NON-PHARMACOLOGICAL METHODS
OF REDUCING PAIN

Many of these have been used successfully with children (Doellman 2003) but they may be used with equal success in adults.

Guided imagery

The patient is asked to imagine places that make them feel relaxed and comfortable to try and alleviate anxiety and fears. Imagery can be used as an adjunct to venepuncture and cannulation and it helps patients cope with the procedure and fosters patient participation, especially when used with relaxation breathing (Courtemanche 1984; Josephson 2004).

Music

This has also been used to reduce the intensity of pain and distress during procedures (Doellman 2003; Capilli *et al.* 2007).

Distraction

Usichenko *et al.* (2004) tested the effectiveness of the cough trick as a method of pain relief during venepuncture. The intensity of the pain during venepuncture was less with it although there was no significant difference with the other variables (hand withdrawal, palm sweating, blood pressure and heart rate). They concluded that it seemed effective but the mechanism remained unclear.

Massage

Wendler (2003) studied the use of the Tellington Touch technique. This is a form of gentle physical touch originally developed for calming of horses. The study reviewed blood pressure (BP), hear rate, anxiety and procedural pain before venepuncture compared with a control group. There was a significant decrease in the touch group in the BP and heart rate, but no other significant differences. However, there were many limitations in the study including the gender and the type of subjects, and the author concluded that the technique needed further study.

Use of transcutaneous electrical nerve stimulation (TENS)
Coyne *et al.* (1995) investigated whether the application of TENS decreased the complaints of pain and unpleasantness with intravenous needle insertion. Their double-blind randomised study was conducted on 71 patients who were placed in one of three groups – placebo TENS, TENS or control. The use of modified brief intense TENS did not produce a reduction in pain (sensory or affective) associated with cannulation, although Lander & Fowler-Kerry (1992) (with children) and Webster *et al.* (1992) (with adults) showed a decrease in procedural pain. The obvious benefits are the lack of long-term side effects or complications but further investigation is required.

PHARMACOLOGICAL METHODS OF REDUCING PAIN

Use of local anaesthetics (LA)
Local anaesthetic agents can help to reduce the pain of venepuncture or cannulation and may lessen the anxiety associated with future procedures involving a needle (Scales 2005). They are widely used in paediatrics and also for anxious adults. They reduce pain but it should be explained to the patient that they will still feel pressure and touch. Any injectable or topical local anaesthetic should only be used upon the written order of a prescriber or under patient group direction (RCN 2010). When the decision is made to use a local anaesthetic, the agent that is the least invasive and/or carries the least risk of allergy should be considered (Moureau & Zonderman 2000; RCN 2010).

Topical local anaesthetics
The contents of any topical local anaesthetics should be left in a small mound and covered with a bio-occlusive dressing. It is not required to spread it as it will spread itself. It is usual practice to apply to more than one potential site in case the first placement fails (Macklin & Chernecky 2004; Lavery & Ingram 2005). The most commonly used local anaesthetic creams are EMLA and Ametop (Dougherty & Watson 2011).

EMLA

Eutectic mixture of local anaesthetics (EMLA) is a cream mixture of two local anaesthetics – lidocaine 2.5% and prilocaine 2.5%. These are emulsified in water and thickened into a cream that becomes oily at room temperature or when applied to the skin (Macklin & Chernecky 2004). The release of the two local anaesthetics into the epidermal and dermal layers of the skin provides anaesthesia and stabilises neuronal membranes by inhibiting the conduction of impulses (Weinstein 2007). Absorption of EMLA is site specific, being more effective on thin epidermal areas than on thick epidermal layers. It is capable of anaesthesia to a maximum depth of 5–6 mm below the skin (Macklin & Chernecky 2004). It takes one hour to be maximally effective (Lavery & Ingram 2005) although some state it should be left on for up to 90 minutes (Patterson *et al.* 2000).

The application is not recommended for patients under 3 months, anyone with known hypersensitivity or use on open areas on skin (Weinstein 2007; Macklin & Chernecky 2004). It is associated with blanching and vasoconstriction and this in turn can result in difficult cannulations (Browne *et al.* 1999). The product comes as a 5 g tube and the recommended application is 2.5 g or half a tube over a small area of skin.

Ametop

Ametop is a topical anaesthetic gel containing amethocaine 4%, xanthan gum, methyl-p-hydroxybenzoate and propyl-p-hydroxybenzoate, water and saline (BNF 2011). It is recommended that it is left on for 30–45 minutes and no longer than 60 minutes. Side effects include erythema (in a third of subjects) oedema and pruritus (Lavery & Ingram 2005). All topical local anaesthetic agents should be removed before venepuncture or cannulation as prolonged skin contact has been associated with skin damage (Hewitt & Scales 1998). Repeated exposure to Ametop has been shown to cause possible red raised areas and blistering in paediatric patients and the site should be observed every 10 minutes (Lavery & Ingram 2005). Browne *et al.* (1999) compared Ametop with EMLA and found that cannulation was less painful using Ametop, and it also caused less vasoconstriction and facilitated easier cannulation.

Intradermal

The intradermal technique is suitable for situations that will not allow the prolonged application time required for creams. It refers to the injection or infiltration of medication around the potential site of the venepuncture or cannulation. The basic goal is to carry out this procedure in order to reduce the level of discomfort of the second needle (or cannula). However, if done improperly the injection can be as painful as inserting a smaller gauge cannula without local anaesthetic (Macklin & Chernecky 2004). The main contraindication is hypersensitivity.

The main benefits are that administering local anaesthetic intradermally is a safe, effective, economical and rapid method of providing local anaesthetic and can be administered immediately prior to the procedure. However, there are some disadvantages and the Infusion Nurses Society (2006) does not recommend its routine use due to the disadvantages such as increased risk of allergic reaction, anaphylaxis and possible inadvertent injection of the drug into the vascular system as well as obliteration of the vein (Weinstein 2007; Dougherty 2008). They state an alternative is to administer an intradermal injection of 0.9% sodium chloride to the side of the vein, which provides an anaesthetic effect but does not increase the patient's risk.

All types of local anaesthetic can be administered but lidocaine is the most common and comes in different concentrations 0.5%, 1% or 2%.

Important factors to reduce the discomfort of intradermal injection are:

- Use small needle, e.g. 25G.
- Ensure local anaesthetic is at room temperature.
- Use only a small amount of local anaesthetic e.g. 0.1–0.3 mL.
- Buffering the lidocaine with bicarbonate can reduce the stinging (Macklin & Chernecky 2004).

Procedure

1. Draw up 0.1 mL of 1% lidocaine in a 1 mL syringe.
2. Insert the needle at a shallow angle (30° or less) next to the vein, about one-third into the skin. The side approach carries

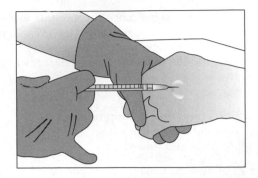

Fig. 10.1 Administering a local anaesthetic. (After Springhouse 2002. Reproduced with permission of Lippincott Williams & Wilkins.)

less risk of accidental vein puncture. If vein is deep it is recommended that the lidocaine is injected over the top of the vein.

3. Always aspirate to check for blood return; if this occurs withdraw the needle and begin the procedure again.
4. Hold thumb on the syringe plunger to avoid unnecessary movement once the needle is under the skin.
5. Inject the lidocaine until a small bleb appears (Fig. 10.1). It may not be necessary to administer the entire amount of the syringe – but the bleb should be the size of a 5p piece.
6. Withdraw the syringe and allow at least 15 seconds for the anaesthetic to work.
7. If the skin wheal seems to obscure the vein, then compress it by massaging the area, and it will disperse. The vein will not be hidden and a small pinprick of blood will still be visible.
8. Insert the needle into the vein (Macklin & Chernecky 2004; Dougherty 2008).

Patterson *et al.* (2000) compared four analgesic agents for pain of application, pain during procedure, cost and convenience. The four agents were:

- EMLA cream
- DCTF (dichlorotetrafluoroethane) spray
- 0.5% lidocaine subcutaneously
- sodium chloride and 0.9% benzyl alcohol subcutaneously.

The authors found no significant difference among the groups for age, sex or difficulty in cannulating. However, there was a significant difference on types of application, with EMLA cream causing no pain and the spray the highest. EMLA was the least convenient to use.

Lidocaine:

- had low pain scores during the procedure
- was low cost and convenient to use
- but was less ideal as it caused pain on application.

However as Brown & Larson (1999) compared cannulation with and without intradermal lidocaine and found that there was significantly lower self-reported pain in the lidocaine group than in the group who did not receive lidocaine, and as a result the authors now offer all patients the choice of having the injection prior to cannulation.

Tetracaine patches
These have been used in infants to achieve effective pain relief and no adverse effects have been reported (Long *et al.* 2003).

Ethyl chloride
Ethyl chloride is a fast acting vapo-coolant spray that provides rapid transient topical anaesthesia for procedures such as venepuncture and cannulation. It has no anaesthetic properties but makes the skin cold and less sensitive as it evaporates, causing instant numbing lasting about 30–45 seconds (Dougherty & Watson 2011).

Iontophoresis
This technique provides analgesia by use of a handheld device with two electrodes using a mild electric current to deliver charged ions of lidocaine 2% and epinephrine 1:100000 solution into the skin. It is effective in 10–20 minutes, has a penetration depth of 10mm, causes minimal discomfort and does not distort the tissues, making it an excellent choice for numbing a site in children and has been shown to be as effective as EMLA (Galinkin *et al.* 2002; Springhouse 2002; Dougherty 2008).

Topical glyceryl trinitrate (GTN)
Topical GTN, 1–2 mg, may also be applied to increase vasodilatation and this in turn may make venepuncture or cannulation easier and therefore less painful (Weinstein 2007).

CONCLUSION
The nurse has an important role to play in ensuring the patient has a positive experience by being honest, forthright and conveying self-assurance (Dougherty 2008). This along with careful patient teaching and a confident, understanding attitude will help patients relax and cooperate (Springhouse 2002).

REFERENCES
Agras, S., Sylvester, D. & Olivean, D. (1969) The epidemiology of common fears and phobias. *Comprehensive Psychiatry*, **10**(2), 151–157.

Ahrens, T., Wiersma, L. & Weilitz, P.B. (1991) Differences in pain perception associated with intravenous catheter insertion. *Journal of Intravenous Nursing*, **14**(2), 85–89.

APA (2000) *Diagnostic and Statistical Manual of Mental Disorders (DSM-IV-TR)*, 4th edn. American Psychiatric Association, Washington DC.

Bennett-Humprey, G. & Boon, C.M.J. (1992) The occurrence of high levels of acute behavioural distress in children and adolescents undergoing routine venepuncture. *Paediatrics*, **90**(1), 87–91.

Berkley, K.J. (1997) Sex differences in pain. *Behavioural and Brain Sciences*, **20**, 371–380.

BNF (2011) *British National Formulary*. BMJ Publishing Group Ltd. London.

Brown, J. & Larson, M. (1999) Pain during insertion of peripheral intravenous catheters with and without intradermal lidocaine. *Clinical Nurse Specialist*, **13**(6), 283–285.

Browne, J., Awad, I., Plant, R., McAdoo, J. & Shorten, G. (1999) Topical amethocaine (Ametop) is superior to EMLA for intravenous cannulation. *Canadian Journal of Anaesthesia*, **46**(11), 1014–1018.

Capilli, S., Anastasi, F., Grotto, R.P., Scotto Abeti, M. & Messeri, A. (2007) Interactive music as a treatment for pain and stress for children during venipuncture: a randomised prospective study. *Journal of Developmental and Behavioral Pediatrics*, **28**(5), 399–403.

Coates, A.S., Abraham, S., Kaye, S.B., *et al.* (1983) On the receiving end: patient perceptions of the side effects of chemotherapy. *European Journal of Cancer Clinical and Oncology*, **19**, 203–208.

Courtemanche, J.B. (1984) Imagery enhances venipuncture. *Journal of Infusion Nursing*, **7**(1), 36.

Coyne, P.J, MacMurren, M., Izzo, T. & Kramer, T. (1995) Transcutaneous electrical nerve stimulator for procedural pain associated with intravenous needlesticks. *Journal of Intravenous Nursing*, **18**(5), 263–267.

Doellman, D. (2003) Pharmacological versus nonpharmacological techniques in reducing venipuncture psychological trauma in pediatric patients. *Journal of Infusion Nursing*, **26**(2), 103–109.

Dougherty, L. (1994) A study to discover how cancer patients perceive the intravenous cannulation experience. Unpublished MSc thesis, University of Surrey, Guildford.

Dougherty, L. (2008) Obtaining peripheral venous access. In: *Intravenous Therapy in Nursing Practice* (eds L. Dougherty & J. Lamb), 2nd edn, pp. 225–270. Blackwell Publishing, Oxford.

Dougherty, L. & Watson, J. (2011) Vascular access devices. In: *The Royal Marsden Hospital Manual of Clinical Nursing Procedures* (eds L. Dougherty & S. Lister), 8th edn. Wiley Blackwell, Oxford.

Ernst, D.J. & Ernst, C. (2001) *Phlebotomy for Nurses and Nursing Personnel*. Healthstar Press, USA.

Feine, J.S., Bushnell, M.C., Miron, D., *et al.* (1991) Sex differences in the perception of noxious heat stimuli. *Pain*, **44**, 255.

Galinkin, J.L, Rose J.B., Harns, K., *et al.* (2002) Lidocaine iontophoresis versus eutectic mixture of local anaesthetics (EMLA) for IV placement in children. *Anesthesia and Analgesia*, **94**(6), 1484–1488.

Griffin, A.M., Butow, P.N., Coates, A.S., *et al.* (1996) On the receiving end. V: Patient perceptions of the side effects of cancer chemotherapy in 1993. *Annals of Oncology*, **7**, 189–195.

Hefler, L., Grimm, C., Leodolter, S. & Tempfer, C. (2004) To butterfly or to needle: the pilot phase. *Annals of Internal Medicine*, **140**(11), 935–936.

Hewitt, T. & Scales, K. (1998) Prolonged contact with topical anaesthetic cream: a case report. *Paediatric Nurse* **10**(2), 22–23.

Infusion Nurses Society (2006) Infusion nursing: standards of practice. *Journal of Infusion Nursing*, **29**(1 Suppl.), S1–S92.

Josephson, D.L. (2004) The delivery, care, maintenance and discontinuation of intravenous infusion therapy. In: *Intravenous Therapy for Nurses: Principles and Practice*, p. 198. Delmar Learning, New York.

Kelley, L., Sklar, D.P, Johnson, D.C. & Tandberg, D. (1997) Women's perceptions of pain and distress during intravenous catheterisation and urethral mini-catheterisation. *American Journal of Emergency Medicine*, **15**(6), 570–572.

Koppel, S. (1999) Treating needle phobia. *Practice Nursing*, **10**(7), 12–13.

Lander, J. & Fowler-Kerry, S. (1992) TENS for children's procedural pain. *Pain*, **52**, 209–216.

Lavery, I. & Ingram, P. (2005) Venepuncture: best practice. *Nursing Standard*, **19**(49), 55–65.

Levine, F.M. & De Simone, L.L. (1991) The effects of experimenter gender on pain report in male and female subjects. *Pain*, **44**, 69–72.

Long, C.P., McCafferty, D.F., Sittlington, N.M., Halliday, H.L., Woolfson, A.D. & Jones, D.S. (2003) Randomized trial of novel tetracaine patch to provide local anaesthesia in neonates undergoing venepuncture. *British Journal of Anaesthesia*, **91**(4), 514–518.

Lücker, P. & Stahlheber-Dilg, B. (2003) Pain related to Optiva 2, Biovalve and Venflon 2 intravenous catheters. *British Journal of Nursing*, **12**(22), 1345–1351.

Macklin, D. & Chernecky, C. (2004) *IV Therapy*. Saunders, St Louis MO.

Miaskowski, C. (1997) Women and pain. *Critical Care Nursing Clinics of North America*, **9**(4), 453–458.

Moureau, N. & Zonderman, A. (2000) Does it always have to hurt? *Journal of Intravenous Nursing*, **23**(4), 213–219.

Otto, M.W. & Dougher, M.J. (1985) Sex differences and personality factors in response to pain. *Perceptual and Motor Skills*, **61**, 383.

Patel, M.X., Baker, D. & Nosarti, C. (2005) Injection phobia: a systematic review of psychological treatments. *Behavioural and Cognitive Psychotherapy*, **33**, 343–349.

Patterson, P., Hussa, A.A., Fedele, K.A. & Hackman, C.M. (2000) Comparison of 4 analgesic agents for venipuncture. *AANA J*, **68**(1), 43–51.

RCN (2010) *Standards for Infusion Therapy*, 3rd edn. Royal College of Nursing, London.

Rogers, P. & Gournay, K. (2001) Phobias: a nature, assessment and treatment. *Nursing Standard*, **15**(30), 37–43.

Scales, K. (2005) Vascular access: a guide to peripheral venous cannulation. *Nursing Standard*, **19**(49), 48–52.

Scales, K. (2008) Anatomy and physiology related to intravenous therapy. In: *Intravenous Therapy in Nursing Practice* (eds L. Dougherty & J. Lamb), 2nd edn, pp. 23–48. Blackwell Publishing, Oxford.

Springhouse (2002) *IV Therapy Made Incredibly Easy*, 2nd edn. Lippincott Williams & Wilkins, Philadelphia.

Stark, M.M. & Brener, N. (2000) Needle phobia. *Journal of Clinical Forensic Medicine*, **7**, 35–38.

Usichenko, T.I., Pavlovic, D., Foellner, S. & Wendt, M. (2004) Reducing venipuncture pain by a cough trick: a randomized crossover volunteer study. *Anesthesia and Analgesia*, **98**, 343–345.

Van den Berg, A.A. & Abeysekera, R.M. (1993) Rationalising venous cannulation: patient factors and lignocaine efficacy. *Anaesthesia*, **48**(1), 84.

Webster, D., Pellegrini, L. & Duffy, K. (1992) Use of transcutaneous electrical nerve stimulation for fingertip analgesia: a pilot study. *Anesthesia and Analgesia*, **21**, 1472–1475.

Weinstein, S. (2007), *Plumer's Principles and Practice of Intravenous Therapy*, 8th edn. Lippincott, Philadelphia.

Wendler, M.C. (2003) Effects of Tellington touch in healthy adults awaiting venipuncture. *Research in Nursing and Health*, **26**, 40–52.

Wilson-Barnett, J. (1976) Patients' emotional reactions to hospitalisation: an exploratory study. *Journal of Advanced Nursing*, **1**, 351–358.

Webliography

- AVA (Association for Vascular Access):
  http://www.avainfo.org/website/article.asp?id=4
- Department of Health (Saving Lives – High Impact interventions from the Department of Health – Cannulation):
  http://www.dh.gov.uk/prod_consum_dh/groups/dh_
  digitalassets/@dh/@en/documents/digitalasset/dh_
  078121.pdf
- Department of Health (The Health Act 2006 – Code of Practice for the Prevention and Control of Health Care Associated Infections):
  http://www.dh.gov.uk/en/Publicationsandstatistics/
  Publications/PublicationsPolicyAndGuidance/DH_4139336
- Infection Prevention Society (incorporating ICNA):
  http://www.ips.uk.net/
- MHRA (Medicines and Healthcare Products Regulatory Agency, UK):
  http://www.mhra.gov.uk/index.htm
- IV Team (intravenous therapy website):
  http://www.ivteam.com/
- Nottingham University ANTT Video:
  http://www.nottingham.ac.uk/nursing/sonet/rlos/placs/
  antt/index.html
- NPSA (National Patient Safety Agency, UK):
  http://www.npsa.nhs.uk/
- RCN (*Standards for Infusion Therapy*):
  http://www.rcn.org.uk/__data/assets/pdf_file/0005/
  78593/002179.pdf
- Structured Learning Programme (Vascular Access Network) Ordering:
  http://veintrain.co.uk
- Transfusion Guidelines and Teaching resources with e-learning packages:
  http://www.transfusionguidelines.org.uk/docs/pdfs/htm_
  edition-4_all-pages.pdf

Venepuncture and Cannulation, first edition. Edited by Sarah Phillips,
Mary Collins and Lisa Dougherty. Published 2011 by Blackwell Publishing Ltd.
© 2011 Blackwell Publishing Ltd.

Glossary

Anti-free-flow administration set: An administration set that stops when removed from the infusion device, yet allows gravity flow when the user manipulates the regulatory mechanism.

Aseptic technique: Mechanisms employed to reduce potential contamination.

Bacteria: Microorganisms that may be non-pathogenic (normal flora) or pathogenic (disease-causing).

Bolus: Concentrated medication and/or solution given rapidly over a short period of time.

Cannula: Hollow tube made of Silastic, rubber, plastic or metal, used for accessing the body.

Catheter: Tube for injecting or evacuating fluids.

Catheter dislodgement: Movement of the catheter into and out of the insertion site. Causes of catheter dislodgement include inappropriate securement of the catheter, and motion of the extremity, neck or shoulder. Catheter dislodgement may cause occlusion of the catheter and lead to a change in the catheter tip location. Signs and symptoms of catheter dislodgement include changes in the external length of the catheter, clinical signs of local catheter infection, and inability to flush or infuse via the catheter.

Chemical incompatibility: Change in the molecular structure or pharmacological properties of a substance that may or may not be visually observed.

Closed system: Administration system with no mechanism for external entry after initial set-up and assembly.

Compatibility: Capability to be mixed and administered without undergoing undesirable chemical and/or physical changes or loss of therapeutic action.

Contamination: Introduction or transference of pathogens or infectious material from one source to another.

Venepuncture and Cannulation, first edition. Edited by Sarah Phillips, Mary Collins and Lisa Dougherty. Published 2011 by Blackwell Publishing Ltd. © 2011 Blackwell Publishing Ltd.

Criteria: Relevant, measurable indicators.

Critical or adverse incident: An event or omission arising during clinical care and causing physical or psychological injury to a patient.

Cross-contamination: Movement of pathogens from one source to another.

Curative: Having healing or remedial properties.

Delivery system: Product that allows for the administration of medication. The system can be integral or can have component parts and includes all products used in the administration, from the solution container to the catheter.

Disinfectant: Agent that eliminates all microorganisms except spores.

Distal: Furthest from the centre or midline of the body or trunk, or furthest from the point of attachment; the opposite of proximal.

Document: Written or printed record containing original, official or legal information.

Documentation: Record in written or printed form, containing original, official or legal information.

Embolus: Mass of undissolved matter present in blood or lymphatic vessel. Embolus may be solid, liquid or gaseous.

Epithelialised: Grown over with epithelial cells; said of a wound or catheter site.

Erythema: Redness of skin along vein track that results from vascular irritation or capillary congestion in response to irritation; may be a precursor to phlebitis.

Extravasation: Inadvertent infiltration of vesicant solution or medication into surrounding tissue; rated by a standard scale.

Extrinsic contamination: Contamination that occurs after the manufacturing process of a product.

Fat emulsion (lipid emulsion): Combination of liquid, lipid and an emulsifying system suitable for intravenous use.

Filter: Special porous device used to prevent the passage of air or other undesired substances; product design determines size of substances retained.

Fluid overload: A fluid and electrolyte imbalance caused by the volume of fluid infusion into a patient.

Free flow: Non-regulated, inadvertent administration of fluid.

Haemolysis: Destruction of the membrane of the red blood cells resulting in the liberation of haemoglobin, which diffuses into the surrounding fluid.

Haemostasis: Arrest of bleeding or of circulation.

Hypertonic: Solution of higher osmotic concentration than that of a reference solution or of an isotonic solution; having a concentration greater than the normal tonicity of plasma.

Hypotonic: Solution of lower osmotic concentration than that of a reference solution or of an isotonic solution; having a concentration less than the normal tonicity of plasma.

Immunocompromised: Having an immune system with reduced capability to react to pathogens or tissue damage.

Incompatible: Incapable of being mixed or used simultaneously without undergoing chemical or physical changes or producing undesirable effects.

Infection: Presence and growth of a pathogenic microorganism.

Infiltration: Inadvertent administration of a non-vesicant solution or medication into surrounding tissue; rated by a standard scale.

Infusate: Parenteral solution administered into the vascular or non-vascular systems; infusion.

Injection access site: Resealable cap or other configuration designed to accommodate needles or needle-less devices for administration of solutions into the vascular system.

Intact system: A closed infusion system.

Intermittent intravenous therapy: Intravenous therapy administered at prescribed intervals with periods of infusion cessation.

Intrinsic contamination: Contamination that occurs during the manufacturing process of a product.

Isolation: Separation of potentially infectious individuals for the period of communicability to prevent or limit direct or indirect transmission of the infectious agent.

Isotonic: Having the same osmotic concentration as the solution with which it is compared (that is, plasma).

Lumen: Interior space of a tubular structure, such as a blood vessel or catheter.

Microorganism: Minute living body not perceptible to the naked eye.

Needle-less system: Substitute for a needle or a sharp access catheter, available in various designs, for example blunt, recessed and valve.

Needlestick injury: Needlestick injuries are wounds caused by needles that accidentally puncture the skin. Needlestick injuries are a hazard for people who work with needles and other sharps equipment. These injuries can occur at any time when people use, handle or dispose of needles. When not disposed of properly, needles can become concealed in linen or waste and injure other workers who encounter them unexpectedly. Needlestick injuries transmit infectious diseases, especially bloodborne viruses.

Non-permeable: Able to maintain integrity.

Non-vesicant: Intravenous medication that generally does not cause tissue damage or sloughing if injected outside a vein.

Occluded: Blocked because of precipitation of infusate, clot formation or anatomic compression.

Osmolality: Characteristic of a solution determined by the ionic concentration of the dissolved substances per unit of solvent; measured in milliosmoles per kilogram.

Osmolarity: Number of osmotically active particles in a solution.

Outcome: Interpretation of documented results.

Palpable cord: Vein that is rigid and hard to the touch.

Palpation: Examination by application of the hands or fingers to the external surface of the body in order to detect evidence of disease or abnormalities in the various organs.

Parenteral: Administered by any route other than the alimentary canal, for example by the intravenous, subcutaneous, intramuscular or mucosal routes.

Parenteral nutrition: Intravenous provision of total nutritional needs for a patient who is unable to take appropriate amounts of food enterally; typical components include carbohydrates, proteins and/or fats, as well as additives such as electrolytes, vitamins and trace elements.

Pathogen: Microorganism or substance capable of producing disease.

Peripherally inserted central catheter (PICC): Soft, flexible, central venous catheter inserted into an extremity and advanced until the tip is positioned in the lower third of the superior vena cava.

pH: Degree of acidity or alkalinity of a substance.

Phlebitis: Inflammation of a vein; may be accompanied by pain, erythema, oedema, streak formation and/or palpable cord; rated by a standard scale.

Phlebotomy: Withdrawal of blood from a vein.

Policy: Written statement describing a course of action; intended to guide decision-making.

Positive pressure: Constant, even force within a catheter lumen that prevents reflux of blood; achieved by clamping while injecting or by withdrawing the needle from the catheter while injecting.

Procedure: Written statement of steps required to complete an action.

Process: Actual performance and observation of performance based on compliance with policies, procedures and professional standards.

Product integrity: Condition of an intact, uncompromised product suitable for intended use.

Proximal: Closest to the centre or midline of the body or trunk, or nearer to the point of attachment; the opposite of distal.

Psychomotor: Characterising behaviours that place primary emphasis on the various degrees of physical skills and dexterity as they relate to the thought process.

Purulent: Containing or producing pus.

Quality assurance/performance improvement: An ongoing, systematic process for monitoring, evaluating and problem solving.

Radiopaque: Impenetrable to X-rays or other forms of radiation; detectable by radiographic examination.

Risk management: Process that centres on identification, analysis, treatment and evaluation of real and potential hazards.

Safety device system: Engineered physical attribute of a device that effectively reduces the risk of bloodborne pathogen exposure.

Scale: Tool to measure gradations.

Sclerosis: Thickening and hardening of the layers in the wall of the vessel.

Semi-quantitative culture technique: Laboratory protocol for isolating and identifying microorganisms.

Sepsis: Presence of infectious microorganisms or their toxins in the bloodstream.

Sharps: Objects in the healthcare setting that can be reasonably anticipated to penetrate the skin and to result in an exposure incident, including but not limited to needle devices, scalpels, lancets, broken glass or broken capillary tubes.

Site protection material: Material used to protect an infusion catheter insertion site.

Standard: Authoritative statement enunciated and promulgated by the profession by which the quality of practice, service or education can be judged.

Standard precautions: Guidelines designed to protect workers with occupational exposure to bloodborne pathogens.

Stylet: Rigid metal object within a catheter designed to facilitate insertion.

Surfactant: Surface-active agent that lowers the surface tension of fluid.

Surveillance: Active, systematic, ongoing observation of the occurrence and distribution of disease within a population and the events or conditions that alter the risk of such occurrence.

Thrombolytic agent: Pharmacological agent capable of dissolving blood clots.

Thrombophlebitis: Inflammation of the vein in conjunction with formation of a blood clot (thrombus).

Thrombosis: Formation, development or existence of a blood clot within the vascular system.

Transfusion therapy: A transfusion consists of the administration of whole blood or any of its components to correct or treat a clinical abnormality.

Transparent semi-permeable membrane (TSM): Sterile, air-permeable dressing that allows visual inspection of the skin surface beneath it; water-resistant.

Vesicant: Agent capable of causing injury when it escapes from the intended vascular pathway into surrounding tissue.

Source: RCN (2010) *Standards for Infusion Therapy*, 3rd edn. RCN, London.

Index

Venepuncture and Cannulation, first edition. Edited by Sarah Phillips,
Mary Collins and Lisa Dougherty. Published 2011 by Blackwell Publishing Ltd.
© 2011 Blackwell Publishing Ltd.